The Editors of **Prevention** *& Jennifer McDaniel, MS, RDN, CSSD, LD*

WITH MARYGRACE TAYLOR

Prevention

MEDITERRANEAN
TABLE

100 Vibrant Recipes to Savor and Share
for Lifelong Health

RECIPES BY THE RODALE TEST KITCHEN

RODALE

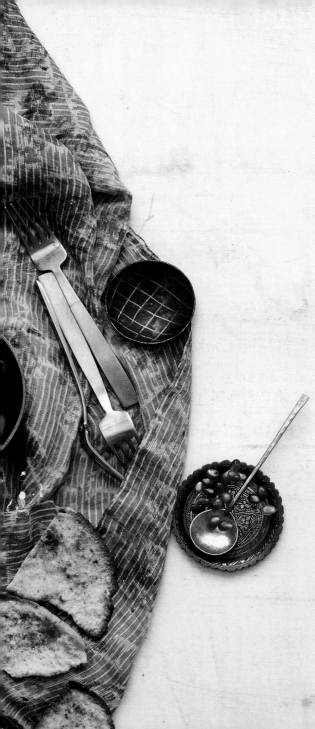

© 2017 by Rodale Inc.
Photographs © 2017 by Rodale Inc.

Rodale books may be purchased for business or promotional use or for special sales. For information, please e-mail: BookMarketing@Rodale.com.

Prevention is a registered trademark of Rodale Inc.

Printed in the United States of America
Rodale Inc. makes every effort to use acid-free ♾, recycled paper ♻.

Food Stylist: Barrett Washburne
Prop Stylist: Paola Andrea
Book design by Yeon Kim
Photographs by Mitch Mandel/Rodale Images

Library of Congress Cataloging-in-Publication Data is on file with the publisher.
ISBN 978–1–63565–022–8 paperback

Distributed to the trade by Macmillan
2 4 6 8 10 9 7 5 3 1   paperback

RODALE

Follow us @RodaleBooks on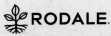

We inspire health, healing, happiness, and love in the world.
Starting with you.

CONTENTS

FOREWORD

Twenty years ago, when I was a senior in high school, my 52-year-old father underwent a quadruple bypass surgery, and it changed my life forever. After experiencing chest pain, my father's doctors discovered his main artery—nicknamed the "widow maker"—was 90 percent blocked. My busy, self-centered teenage life came to a halt. I faced the fact that I could lose my dad. Dad's surgery was successful, and it brings me joy to say that my three sons have a grandfather, but that experience planted the seed that grew into my decision to become a dietitian. I believe in the power of prevention and our ability to influence our health, one forkful at a time.

While most of us know that diet plays a role in our health, we don't always act on that knowledge. About 80 percent of chronic diseases, including obesity, heart disease, and diabetes, could be prevented with a healthy lifestyle. Every meal and snack is an opportunity to support our short- and long-term health, and yet 7 out of 10 deaths per year are due to chronic disease. In my private practice, clients frequently come to me confused and mislead by mixed messages the health world often conveys. Should they follow this or that diet? Do they need a "bad foods" vs. "good foods" list? Should they cut entire food groups?

The truth is that they yearn for sound nutrition advice that is flexible, realistic, and proven over time. I prefer this, too. I would rather discuss nourishment and fuel, not calorie counting and nutrient categorization. If there is one way of eating or lifestyle in line with those philosophies, it is the Mediterranean diet.

I became interested in the Mediterranean diet through my research into longevity. It was clear that individuals in the Mediterranean region, in places such as Greece, Crete, Spain, Italy, Tunisia, Syria, Portugal, France, Morocco, and Lebanon, not only lived longer than Americans but also lived with less disease. What was it about the Mediterranean way that supported a high-quality, long life? It wasn't hard to find the evidence. The Mediterranean diet has been the subject of thousands of studies, making it one of the most studied ways of eating. Researchers confirm that the native diet of the Mediterranean region lowers the risk of inflammatory-related diseases. Also, shifting from the standard American diet to the Mediterranean diet improves health and lowers disease risk. It has the power to both prevent *and* treat.

The Mediterranean diet has been the foundation of my diet and lifestyle advice, with everyday foods including olive oil, fruits, vegetables, beans, nuts, whole grains, and herbs and weekly servings of fish, poultry, and dairy foods. My clients embrace a satisfying, healthy-fat diet rich in nuts, seeds, and olive oil. Abundant, creative use of spices and herbs adds flavor and variety in place of less healthy go-to seasonings like butter, added salt, and sugar. This diet celebrates a variety of foods as opposed to a black-and-white list that tells you to "eat this, not that." Even meat has a place—it just isn't the center of attention. The flexibility of the diet makes it easy to incorporate into anyone's unique eating style.

The simple and flavorful ingredients will make you want to linger and savor your meal.

It is my hope that you not only reap the benefits of the diet but also slow down and mindfully enjoy these meals with friends and family. The Mediterranean way is not rushed, emphasizing community, connection, and celebration above all else.

Over the years, I have looked for a cookbook to recommend to my clients to make it easy to adopt the Mediterranean diet. Our team at *Prevention* magazine has created the perfect compilation of Mediterranean recipes for every meal, and you can trust that the recipes are not only nutritious but also representative of the tastes and flavors of the Mediterranean region.

Come to our Mediterranean table. Make the choice to put more of these beneficial and delicious foods on your plate and build a long, healthy life.

Jennifer McDaniel, MS, RDN, CSSD, LD

ACKNOWLEDGMENTS

I owe many thanks and appreciation to the following special people:

My husband, PJ, for being an adventurous eater. He takes my good meals with the bad ones and never complains. More importantly, he helps me raise three healthy eaters. Smiling while he eats his veggies means the world to me. My mom, Jj, for teaching me at a young age how to cook and for allowing me to experiment and play in the kitchen. Watching her drink the leftover water from cooked broccoli taught me early that "food is thy medicine." No nutrients should be wasted! My dad, Doug, for believing and supporting his foodie daughter even though he is a "meat and potatoes" kind of guy. Dad's endorsement will forever keep me motivated to work hard and pursue my passions. My sister, Erin, for being my number-one cheerleader. Her unwavering support means more than she will ever know. Marygrace and the team from *Prevention,* for selecting me as your nutrition expert for this cookbook. I have learned and benefited from their guidance and expertise.

—*Jennifer McDaniel*

To our fantastic editor, Allison Janice, for her smart, insightful direction and thoughtful guidance, and Jennifer McDaniel, for her collaboration and commitment to making this book a truly valuable resource for our readers.

Thanks also to Rodale's test kitchen for developing healthy, creative, and truly delicious recipes. Most important, thanks to my husband, Sam Taylor, for his constant support, patience, and encouragement.

—*Marygrace Taylor*

INTRODUCTION

Welcome to the Table!

If you've been searching for a fresh, uncomplicated style of eating that nourishes your body, your heart, and your soul, you've come to the right place. The countries bordering the Mediterranean Sea have long been known for their simple, deeply satisfying cuisine and their relaxed, family-oriented approach to mealtime. The Mediterranean diet isn't just delicious—it's a warm, inviting change of pace from the nonstop chaos that many of us are used to.

That alone might be enough to have you saying, "Pass the olive oil!" but there's more—and it's important. Following a Mediterranean diet just might be one of the very best things that you can do for your health. Countless studies that have collectively researched and surveyed thousands of people show that eating Mediterranean-style could significantly lower your risk for chronic diseases, including heart disease, diabetes, some cancers, and Alzheimer's disease. This diet can also help you reach or maintain a healthy weight without counting calories, cutting out entire food groups, or following complicated rules.

To be clear, the Mediterranean diet isn't a *diet* in the self-denying, sacrificing sense of the word. Instead, it's a lifestyle approach to eating rooted in a centuries-old tradition of using fresh, high-quality ingredients to make home-cooked meals that are shared in the company of family and friends. The word *diet* itself actually stems from the Greek word *diaita*, which has been translated as "way of living" or "habits and customs of the body."[1]) Just look at the millions of people in Greece, Italy, Spain, Turkey, Morocco, and the other countries surrounding the Mediterranean Sea who continue to eat in this simple and rewarding way, even as America's fast-food, drive-thru lifestyle has taken hold. The Mediterranean diet's staying power is a testament to its inherent value—and the science-backed benefits have never been clearer.

So grab a seat, and make yourself comfortable. In this book, you'll discover the latest research on how the Mediterranean diet can transform your health and well-being. You'll also learn what it truly means to eat Mediterranean, plus you'll find suggestions and advice for turning everyday meals into family-focused experiences to savor together. And, of course, you'll find over 100 fresh, mouthwatering recipes for Mediterranean-inspired breakfasts, salads, soups, sandwiches, snacks, sides, dinners, and desserts, along with menu ideas for every occasion—from quick weekday lunches to weekend brunches and family dinners. It all begins here, at *Prevention Mediterranean Table*.

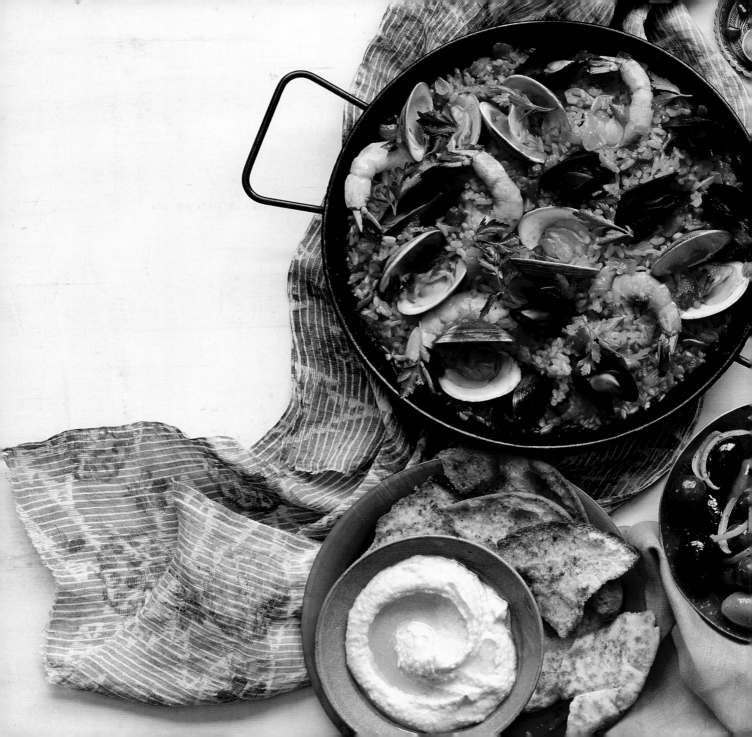

PART I

The FOOD and the LIFESTYLE

Chapter 1
The Power of Going Mediterranean

Chances are you've seen articles and reports highlighting the many benefits of the Mediterranean diet at least a few times over the years. Now more than ever, this traditional style of eating is being touted for its healthfulness as diet trends come and go and people search for a style of eating that fits into their everyday lives, and for good reason.

An ever-growing body of evidence shows that a Mediterranean-style diet is one of the most effective ways to reach a healthy weight, feel great, and live a long, vigorous life. It's also one of the most appetizing and indulgent—allowing for pastas, cheeses, and even dessert in moderation, not to mention wine. The Mediterranean diet has long been beloved for its deliciousness, its simplicity, and its ability to bring families together over food. And in a world where confusion over healthy eating and the best diets for losing weight—from the standard low-carb, low-fat diets and calorie counting to the more recent gluten-free, paleo, and vegan trends—and hectic, time-strapped schedules reign supreme, it might be just what you're looking for.

So what exactly does it mean to eat Mediterranean, and what can this ancient diet do for you and your family? Let's find out.

WHAT *IS* THE MEDITERRANEAN DIET?

In the late 1950s, physiologist and dietary researcher Ancel Keys was conducting

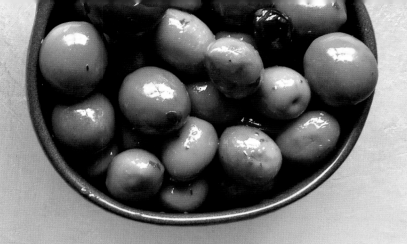

research in southern Italy and Greece's island of Crete when he happened upon a surprising discovery: The people who lived in this warm, sunny paradise seemed healthier than all of the other populations he'd studied around the globe—including places like the United States, Japan, the Netherlands, and Yugoslavia. In fact, the people of the Mediterranean enjoyed some of the longest life spans and the lowest rates of heart disease in the world.

Other experts might have wondered whether the benefits came from the abundance of golden sunshine, fresh air, or invigorating salt water—all things that the Mediterranean region is celebrated for. But Keys had a different theory. What if the impressive health boost was actually coming from the *food*? At the time, the suggestion

that what we eat could have such a significant impact on our health and longevity was considered radical. But looking back, Keys' light bulb moment would set the stage for much of what we know about nutrition today. Including the fact that following a Mediterranean-style diet is one of the best things you can do for your health—and your well-being.

Since then, this theory has been proven by countless studies, including a 5-year study of nearly 8,000 adults, which concluded that following a Mediterranean diet rich in olive oil and nuts could reduce the risk for heart disease by as much as 30 percent.[1] Another that looked at nearly 25,000 adults found that eating Mediterranean-style is linked to lower levels of inflammatory markers that could raise the risk for disease, along with

4

improved levels of blood sugar, blood pressure, and unhealthy fats in the blood.[3]

▌VARIATIONS ON A THEME

Ancel Keys saw that the people living in the countries that border the Mediterranean Sea had many of their own distinctive dishes and recipes. But stepping back to see the bigger picture, he noticed that the diets of these rich and diverse cultures all shared a similar pattern: They were based largely around fresh fruits and vegetables, whole grains, and beans. These cultures used olive oil (and plenty of it) as their primary fat and ate generous amounts of nuts and seeds. They flavored their food using herbs and spices instead of salt. They enjoyed fresh seafood, yogurt and cheese, and red wine several times a week. And they ate very little meat, refined carbohydrates, or processed foods.[4]

Though Keys may have been the first researcher to document the Mediterranean diet's potent health effects, the people living in the coastal regions of southern Europe and Northern Africa had been eating this way since, well, since there were humans populating these regions. The warm, sunny climate made it ideal for growing an abundance of fruits and vegetables, including olives that could be used to make olive oil. Fresh seafood was plentiful and easy to catch. Meat and poultry were saved for special occasions, since slaughtering a cow or chicken meant it could no longer produce valuable milk or eggs. And whole grains were less laborious to produce than their refined counterparts, which required processing to strip them of their nutrient-rich outer hulls. For the Mediterranean people, eating a traditional diet of wholesome, minimally processed foods was the only option available for most of history. It just took until the 20th century for science to catch up to nature and identify that it's the best option for health and well-being for all humans.

Of course, the Mediterranean region is vast and diverse. How could the millions of people living in 18 different countries—from Italy to Greece to Turkey to Morocco to Spain—possibly all eat the same way? The answer is, they don't! Throughout the Mediterranean, you'll find different dishes and dietary staples from one country to the next, with plenty of local variations from region to region—and even from village to village. *Diet* might be a convenient word to use, but the Mediterranean diet is really a bigger, broader style of eating that emphasizes certain foods over others. The recipes in this book all follow the basic tenets of the diet while also borrowing from the different food cultures and traditions from around the area.

It's also more than just a collection of healthy foods. The Mediterranean diet is a way of life—and if you're one of the millions of Americans who have tried to lose weight or improve their health with complicated or restrictive eating plans, you'll find it *really* refreshing. Above all, the Mediterranean diet values the deep satisfaction that comes from eating fresh, delicious meals. Especially when they're enjoyed with others. As far as Mediterranean culture is concerned, food is meant to be shared with the people you care about—not eaten in the car on the way to dropping off the kids at school before work, at a desk while checking e-mails, with the kids constantly checking their phones, or alone in front of the

5

>>> Your Mediterranean Menu

Just how much of these foods should you aim to eat on a daily or weekly basis? To make your diet truly Mediterranean—and reap the impressive benefits that come with it—here's what you should aim for.[5]

DAILY	SEVERAL TIMES A WEEK	OCCASIONALLY
Fruits and vegetables	Fish and shellfish (at least twice weekly)	Red or processed meat
Whole grains	Eggs	Butter
Olive oil	Cheese	Refined grains
Beans and legumes	Yogurt	Sweets and desserts
Nuts and seeds	Poultry	Soda and sugary drinks
Herbs and spices	Red wine	Packaged or highly processed snacks

TV. After all, preparing even simple meals takes work and time. And that effort is worth savoring and celebrating more often.

Of course, the idea of a whole new style of eating might seem a little overwhelming. Questions like "Can I still have my favorite snacks?" and "Do I need to clean out my pantry?" and "A peaceful meal? In my house?" are probably on your mind. But once you learn some more about how adopting a Mediterranean-style diet can help you get more pleasure out of your meals while seriously boosting your health *and* helping you reach a healthier weight, you'll be

hooked—and you'll see how easy eating Mediterranean can be. It all starts with learning just how powerful this diet really is.

THE SCIENCE-BACKED BENEFITS

More than 60 years after Ancel Keys first noticed the Mediterranean diet's positive health impacts, it has become one of the most well-studied eating patterns in the world. And the findings are truly staggering. Today, we know that many of the individual foods that form the diet's base serve up valuable benefits.

But when you take a step back to look at the bigger picture, there's this: Mounting evidence suggests that the Mediterranean diet, when enjoyed as a whole, just might be one of the healthiest styles of eating in the world. In a 2014 analysis of eight different dietary approaches (including low-carb, low-fat, vegan, and paleo diets), researchers concluded that minimally processed, plant-based diets, like the Mediterranean diet, are the best at protecting health and preventing disease.[6] (Some experts have even described it as "very close to if not the ideal diet."[7]) Here are some of the important ways that a Mediterranean diet can help you.

YOU'LL PROTECT YOUR HEART AND LOWER YOUR CHOLESTEROL

When it comes to eating for heart health, the evidence is clear: Eating a Mediterranean-style diet can dramatically reduce your risk for heart disease or stroke. One British study following some 25,000 healthy adults for more than a decade found that those who stuck more closely to a Mediterranean diet were up to 16 percent less likely to develop heart disease compared to those who followed other diets.[8] Another, which analyzed the diets of some 15,000 adults who already had heart disease, found that the more Mediterranean the participants ate, the less likely they were to have a heart attack, stroke, or heart-related death.[9]

Why? A Mediterranean-style eating

›› Where's the Pizza?

If you're like most Americans, when you hear about Greek or Italian food, you might think of gyros or eggplant Parmesan. After all, that's probably the kind of fare served at most restaurants near you! But in fact, many of these classic dishes were invented right here in America or were heavily modified to please US palates. And though American-style eating habits are becoming more common in the Mediterranean (and around the world), most home cooks—along with the Italian cafés, Spanish tapas bars, or Greek tavernas—still tend to stick with tradition. Instead of heaping piles of spaghetti and meatballs, you'll find vegetable-heavy meals with smaller quantities of fish or poultry. Pastas are lightly sauced, not smothered. And when pizza *does* show up, it's typically the size of a plate—not a car tire.

7

pattern lowers levels of LDL, or "bad," cholesterol while keeping levels of HDL, or "good," cholesterol high. Trading unhealthy saturated fats found in red meat for generous quantities of healthy monounsaturated ones—like olive oil and nuts—helps prevent the buildup of artery-clogging bad cholesterol. Many Mediterranean-style foods, like olive oil, are also thought to promote healthy blood vessel function, which helps keep blood pressure in check and lowers the risk for stroke. The copious amounts of fiber- and antioxidant-rich fruits and vegetables and the use of whole grains over processed refined grains also provide heart-healthy benefits—especially now that we know processed grains can increase the risk of heart disease.

Some findings even go as far as to suggest that eating Mediterranean could be more beneficial for protecting heart health than some prescription medications. Among high-risk people, eating a Mediterranean diet could potentially reduce the risk of cardiovascular events like heart attack or stroke by a whopping 30 percent, according to a study published in the *New England Journal of Medicine*.[10] Compare that to cholesterol-lowering medications called statins, which have been shown to lower the risk of heart problems by around 24 percent,[11] while serving up possible side effects like muscle pain,

> >>> **Going Backward**
> The Mediterranean diet doesn't just help prevent diseases from happening in the first place. Some research[12] even suggests that in the long term, following a Mediterranean-style diet can help *reverse* metabolic syndrome—a cluster of conditions such as obesity, hyperglycemia, and hypertension that raise the risk for heart disease, stroke, and diabetes. Now, *that's* a powerful prescription.

as well as liver damage and increased blood sugar. Of course, decisions over managing your heart health are best discussed with your doctor. But eating a healthy diet *does* seem a whole lot nicer than popping a pill, doesn't it?

YOU'LL LOSE WEIGHT— AND KEEP IT OFF

If you're looking to get leaner, there are countless diets out there that promise to help. But eating Mediterranean might be the best, most enjoyable way to reach your goal—and *stay* there for good. In an *American Journal of Medicine* review of five studies that pitted the Mediterranean diet against other weight-loss methods over a period of 12 months,

8

Mediterranean-style diets were found to help people lose more weight than low-fat ones. Eating Mediterranean was also just as effective as other restrictive weight-loss methods, like cutting carbs or avoiding sugar.[13] In short, it delivered the same results or better—*without* the dieters having to give up great flavor or entire food groups.

And you don't have to worry about tallying up calories. Though it's important to pay attention to portion size and hunger levels and indulge in moderation, findings suggest that you don't need to get caught up in the numbers game when you eat Mediterranean. In a 5-year study of nearly 7,500 adult participants—most of whom were overweight—those who followed a Mediterranean-style diet *without* counting calories lost more weight and shed more belly

fat than those who stuck to a low-fat diet.[16]

Perhaps most significantly, a Mediterranean-style diet is easy to stick to, and not just because you don't have to bother breaking out the calculator at every meal. The emphasis on fresh flavors and healthy fats means that everything you eat is satisfying and flavorful, so you won't feel deprived. What's more, it's easy to find Mediterranean-style options *anywhere*, from fish and roasted vegetables at a restaurant to yogurt and fresh fruit at the airport to hummus, olives, and a wedge of cheese at a cocktail party. Add it all up, and you can see how losing weight—and keeping it off—the Mediterranean way is both easy and truly enjoyable.

YOU'LL REDUCE YOUR RISK FOR CHRONIC DISEASES

A healthier heart and trimmer waistline are just the start of the many benefits the Mediterranean diet has to offer. Eating a diet rich in fruits and vegetables, whole grains, fish, and healthy fats packs an antioxidant, anti-inflammatory punch that research shows can play a role in preventing a plethora of serious ailments, like these:

• **TYPE 2 DIABETES.** Because eating a fiber-rich Mediterranean diet promotes a healthy weight and stable blood sugar levels, it could

>>> **22 pounds**
That's how much weight you could lose in a year just by following a Mediterranean-style diet, suggests one *American Journal of Medicine* study.[14] Kids can reap the benefits, too. Findings suggest that children who eat a Mediterranean diet are 15 percent less likely to become overweight or obese.[15]

help you avoid type 2 diabetes. In fact, one review in the journal Metabolism that looked at nearly 137,000 adults concluded that sticking closely to a Mediterranean diet can slash type 2 diabetes risk by an incredible 23 percent.[17]

• **CANCER.** Experts have long noticed that cancer rates are lower in countries bordering the Mediterranean Sea than in the United States or in northern Europe. And, indeed, research has shown that eating a Mediterranean-style diet is linked to lower rates of colorectal, breast, stomach, prostate, liver, and head and neck cancers, found a *Current Nutrition Reports* review.[18] One small study of cancer survivors even showed that Mediterranean diets could help stop certain types of cancer—like breast cancer—from coming back.[19]

• **COGNITIVE DECLINE.** A Mediterranean-style diet can even give your brain a boost. Experts have recently discovered that older adults who eat this way experience less of the normal age-related brain shrinkage that can affect learning and memory.[20] So it might not come as much of a surprise to learn that eating a Mediterranean-style diet could slash the risk for Alzheimer's disease by as much as 53 percent[21] and even *improve* your long- and short-term memory, research shows.[22]

YOU JUST MIGHT LIVE A LONGER, HAPPIER LIFE

When you think about all of the serious health conditions that can potentially be averted by following a Mediterranean-style diet, it's no wonder that eating this way could help you live longer. An 8-year study of some 23,000 Greek adults found that sticking closely to a Mediterranean diet was linked to 14 percent lower risk of dying from any cause.[23]

And, indeed, Mediterranean regions like Ikaria, Greece, and Sardinia, Italy, have some of the largest concentrations of centenarians—people who are age 100 or older—in the world.

It seems that the Mediterranean diet has the incredible ability to slow down the rate at which the body's cells age. Recent Harvard research shows that people who eat Mediterranean-style actually have longer telomeres—caps at the end of each strand of DNA that protect the chromosomes.[24] Everyone's telomeres get shorter with age, which increases the risk for age-related diseases like heart disease and cancer. And while high levels of oxidative stress and inflammation can cause telomeres to get shorter faster, the antioxidant and anti-inflammatory compounds found in a Mediterranean diet seem to play a role in keeping our telomeres longer for, well, longer.

Another important reason why eating Mediterranean could lead to a longer life: A Mediterranean diet can have a positive impact on your mood and emotional health. Loading up on highly processed, sugary foods is linked to higher rates of anxiety and depression, while eating mostly whole, unprocessed foods seems to have the opposite effect.[25]

In fact, there is some research to suggest that eating Mediterranean can lead to significant improvements in mood among people with severe depression.[26] Sharing meals, a common practice among Mediterranean eaters, is thought to promote stronger relationships, too (more on that in Chapter 3).[27] And people with stronger social ties tend to be happier than those who feel isolated.[28]

That's important, because happiness is the key to health. Many experts believe that chronic negative emotions, like stress, anger, and anxiety, are toxic to the body—increasing inflammation and upping the risk for serious health problems like heart disease and diabetes. Having an optimistic attitude, on the other hand, is linked to a lower risk of chronic disease—which could translate to a longer, healthier life.[29]

INGREDIENTS FOR HEALTH

At this point, we've talked about the impressive health benefits that come with eating a Mediterranean diet, but what makes this style of eating so potent when it comes to your health, your weight, and your overall well-being? The foods that form the backbone of the Mediterranean diet deliver impressive benefits on their own. But they become even *more* powerful when you eat them together. Enjoying them in the right proportions is important, too. Chances are you already cook with olive oil or occasionally have fish and vegetables for dinner. But shifting toward an eating pattern where you have these kinds of foods *most* of the time can add up to big changes for your health.

So what foods should you have on a daily or weekly basis, and how can they help you? What foods should you enjoy less often— saving those for once in a while? Read on

▌ EVERYDAY FOODS

Day-to-day Mediterranean-style eating can be summed up in one word: *Plants*. Mounting evidence shows that plant-heavy eating patterns, like the Mediterranean diet, pack the biggest health punch—even more so than

11

12

trendy paleo and low-carb diets, according to Yale University nutrition experts writing in the *Annual Review of Public Health*.[30] From fresh salads to whole grain pilafs to hearty stuffed vegetables and bean soups, plant foods like those listed below show up in virtually every Mediterranean meal, every day.

• **WHOLE GRAINS,** like whole grain bread or pita, whole wheat pasta, brown rice, quinoa, oatmeal, and bulgur wheat

• **VEGETABLES,** like leafy greens, root vegetables (e.g., carrots and beets), winter squash, tomatoes, broccoli, cauliflower, green beans, asparagus, zucchini and summer squash, onions and garlic, white potatoes and sweet potatoes, and fresh herbs

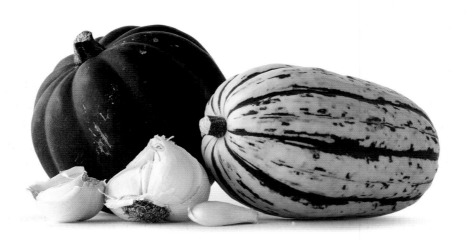

- **FRUIT,** like berries, citrus fruits, apples, pears, pomegranates, apricots, peaches, plums, figs, and dates
- **OLIVE OIL,** along with other healthy plant-based fats, like olives and avocado
- **BEANS AND LEGUMES,** like chickpeas, lentils, split peas, white beans, and kidney beans
- **NUTS AND SEEDS,** like walnuts, almonds, pistachios, sesame seeds, and tahini (sesame seed butter)
- **RED WINE** once daily, if you'd like

An abundance of these plant-based foods means that the Mediterranean diet is considerably higher in fiber than the Standard American Diet—also referred to as SAD. You won't find much roughage on a plate of a burger and fries! That's important, because fiber makes the digestive system more efficient, promotes gut health by helping to grow and maintain gut microbiota in the intestines, and steadies blood sugar levels so you stay satisfied for longer and are less likely to crave sugary junk.

And that's just the beginning. The fiber in a Mediterranean diet also acts like a magnet to grab onto cholesterol particles in your bloodstream and move them out of your body quickly, so they're less able to clog your arteries. Fiber also nourishes the good bacteria in your gut, which in turn, produce short-chain fatty acids thought to promote heart health,

> ### ››› Don't Resist the Starch!
>
> One more reason to love Mediterranean-style sources of complex carbs: Many of them, including barley, oats, lentils, and split peas, are naturally rich in resistant starch, a unique fiberlike starch. Because it's indigestible and cannot be absorbed, resistant starch delivers fewer calories than other types of carbohydrates while taking up more space in the digestive system. What's more, research suggests that resistant starch can boost fat burning[31] as well as set off the release of fullness-signaling hormones,[32] both of which could help you lose more weight. Other Mediterranean staples, including pasta and potatoes, become *higher* in resistant starch after they're cooked and cooled, and even after reheating.

reduce the risk for diabetes, and fight inflammation that can raise the risk for other chronic diseases.[33] A warm grain and bean salad or a heaping pile of greens might sound pretty good with a side of some serious heart health.

Plants serve up plenty of beneficial antioxidants called phytonutrients, as well. Plants use phytonutrients to protect themselves from

>>> Plant Power

Pass the greens, please! On average, plant foods, like fruits, vegetables, nuts, and beans, pack around 64 times more phytonutrients than animal-based ones, like meat or dairy, according to *Nutrition Journal* research.[34] Loading up on a variety of plants will help you get a wide range of these powerful antioxidants, but the following picks are especially potent.[35] Get some colors on your plate, and aim to eat them as often as you can!

❖ **Dark red and purple plant foods,** including berries, cherries, red cabbage, black plums and prunes, and black beans and kidney beans, are top sources of anthocyanins, antioxidant compounds thought to support heart and brain health, fight obesity and diabetes, and potentially reduce the risk for some cancers.[36]

❖ **Dark leafy greens,** like kale, spinach, and Swiss chard, are rich in vitamin C, which may help fight diabetes, heart disease, and cancer.[37] They also contain lutein and zeaxanthin, which can promote eye health and help reduce the risk for cataracts and age-related macular degeneration.[38]

❖ **Bell peppers** are another top source of vitamin C. They also serve up beta-carotene, which is linked to lower rates of metabolic syndrome.[39]

❖ **Apples and artichokes** are loaded with quercetin, a flavonoid that some findings suggest could boast anticancer properties. Quercetin is also thought to lower blood pressure and promote healthy cholesterol.[40]

❖ **Walnuts** contain almost twice as many antioxidants as an equivalent amount of other nuts, according to University of Scranton research. Namely polyphenols, which are thought to boost heart heath.[41]

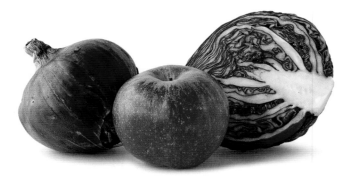

stressors in their environments, and when we eat them, *we* get that same protection—from things like the sun's UV rays and pollutants in the air to the refined sugar and additives found in many processed foods. That translates to lower levels of inflammation and cell damage in the body, which can help reduce the risk for chronic diseases like heart disease, cancer, and Alzheimer's disease. Fruits and vegetables, along with herbs, spices, and red wine, are all top phytonutrient sources—and the more of these foods you eat, the more protection you get.

Finally, there's healthy, monounsaturated fat—found in foods like olive oil, nuts, and seeds. Throughout the Mediterranean, folks tend to get anywhere from 30 to 40 percent of their calories from fat, estimate experts.[42] Which might sound like a lot, especially if you remember the days when fat was feared above all else (there are still low-fat and no-fat versions of all sorts of popular products).

But a growing body of research shows that monounsaturated fat doesn't just *not* make you fat—it can actually help you to stay lean and protect your heart. It also seems to work in harmony with fruits and vegetables by enhancing the absorption of important nutrients. Plus, it simply makes food taste good!

▮ WEEKLY FOODS

Plant foods might be the stars of the Mediterranean diet, but animal products play an essential supporting role. Occasionally, they're the main component of the meal, like Olive Oil–Poached Fish over Citrus Salad (page 194) or the yogurt in the Mediterranean Muesli and Breakfast Bowl (page 86). But more often, they're enjoyed in smaller quantities to make meals even more mouthwatering, like some cheese sprinkled on top of a green salad or a bit of shredded chicken stirred into a vegetable and bean soup. Consider these foods your good-for-you accents. Aim to eat fish and shellfish at least twice weekly, and enjoy moderate helpings of the other foods a few times a week (or less often, if you'd like).

- **FISH,** like salmon, tuna, herring, black cod, sardines, and anchovies
- **SHELLFISH,** like mussels, oysters, clams, and shrimp
- **EGGS**—yes, the white *and* the yolk!
- **DAIRY** like fat-free or 1% milk and low-fat plain yogurt
- **FLAVORFUL, FULL-FAT CHEESES,** like Parmesan, Manchego, feta, Halloumi, and ricotta, in small quantities
- **POULTRY,** like chicken or turkey

Traditionally, folks in the Mediterranean tended to choose fish, eggs, dairy, and poultry over red or processed meat because they were just more economical. But now, experts know that these protein sources serve up serious benefits. Most notably, seafood is a top source of omega-3 fatty acids, essential fats that most Americans don't get enough of. They're best known for protecting heart health by lowering blood pressure, boosting blood vessel function, lowering levels of bad cholesterol, and fighting inflammation. In fact, a Mayo Clinic review found that consumption of omega-3-rich foods was tied to a 16 percent lower risk of heart disease in people with overly high levels of bad fat or cholesterol in their blood.[43] Omega-3s have also been shown to reduce the risk for breast and colon cancer, help prevent Alzheimer's disease and dementia, ease symptoms of rheumatoid arthritis, and fight depression.

As for dairy, you might remember back to the fat-phobic 1980s and 1990s, when anything other than rubbery fat-free cheese or skim milk was seen as a heart attack on a plate or in a glass. But more recent research shows that followers of the Mediterranean diet—with their fatty cheeses and yogurt—were right all along. Not only do full- and low-fat dairy foods *not* raise the risk for heart disease[44]—they may actually help lower it while delivering other important benefits.

People who eat full-fat dairy are no more likely to develop heart disease or type 2 diabetes than those who go fat-free, according to a review published in the *European Journal of Nutrition*.[45] At the same time, they tend to weigh less and are less likely to gain weight over time. There's also the fact that foods like yogurt and cheese contribute to healthy gut bacteria[46]—which play a role in everything from digestive health to immunity to lower levels of artery-clogging fat in the blood.

It's a similar story for eggs. Despite those dire, outdated warnings to stick with just the whites, the cholesterol in foods like egg yolks has a much smaller effect on heart health than unhealthy fats. Not only does an egg a day *not* raise cholesterol in healthy adults—eggs are actually a rich source of heart-protecting nutrients, like vitamins B_{12} and D, riboflavin, and folate. Plus, the protein in eggs can support your weight-loss efforts by keeping you fuller for longer, so you're less tempted to snack on junk between meals.

▌ OCCASIONAL FOODS

Remember that delicious food is one of life's pleasures—and it should make you feel good. Most of the time, that means enjoying the tasty, powerful foods we just talked about. But there's room for a little bit of *everything*

››› Choosing Safer Seafood

Fish and shellfish are some of the healthiest proteins out there, but seafood can also contain toxins like mercury and polychlorinated biphenyls (PCBs), which are linked to cancer and birth defects.[47] Follow these tips to find—and serve—the cleanest options.

⁂ **Feast on smaller fish and shellfi'sh.** Fish like shark, swordfish, tilefish, and king mackerel are larger and therefore tend to accumulate the most toxins. Steer clear of those, and instead choose wild Pacific salmon, farmed rainbow trout, US wild-caught or farmed shrimp, US farmed tilapia, Pacific halibut or cod, sardines or anchovies, and US farmed oysters, mussels, or clams. They're smaller and cleaner.

⁂ **Be a savvy shopper.** Ask your fishmonger for specific information about where your seafood is from (domestic is better than imported) or how it was caught or farmed (farmed fish should be raised sustainably, without antibiotics). For more guidelines you can take on the go, consider downloading Food & Water Watch's pocket guide for choosing smart seafood, available at foodandwaterwatch.org.

⁂ **Cook it clean.** Pollutants tend to accumulate in a fish's fat, so opt for cooking methods that allow excess fat to drain away, recommends the Environmental Defense Fund.[48] Broiling, grilling, and poaching are all healthy options.

⁂ **Know the truth about tuna.** A great source of dietary protein, omega-3 fatty acids, iodine, iron, and B vitamins—tuna is very common and a great fish to eat on the Mediterranean diet. Be careful, however, because eating too much canned tuna may pose health risks, especially for pregnant women, breastfeeding women, and young children, as it contains varying amounts of methylmercury—a known neurotoxin. Canned tuna can contain high levels of sodium, so limit your consumption to a few times per week only. Also be sure to choose canned light tuna over canned white/albacore tuna, as it contains less mercury.

in a Mediterranean-style diet. You don't have to kiss things like red meat, sugary desserts, or refined carbohydrates like white bread or white pasta goodbye completely. You just need to have them less often.

Instead of every day or every week, treat yourself a few times a month. Going heavy on foods that are high in saturated fat—from burgers to baked goods—can raise the risk for heart disease. But swapping just 1 percent of the saturated fats in your diet for unsaturated fats, whole grains, or plant proteins like beans can *reduce* heart disease risk by up to 8 percent, found a recent *British Medical Journal* analysis of 116,000 people.[49] It's also worth limiting your consumption of packaged or highly processed foods—foods that are significantly changed from their natural state.[50] (For instance, fresh strawberries have to go through a high level of processing to become strawberry fruit gummies.) These foods tend to be higher in sugary, refined carbs that can increase levels of unhealthy fats in the blood, promote the buildup of belly fat, and cause unhealthy blood sugar spikes that can raise the risk for diabetes. They're also more likely to contain artificial ingredients or additives, some of which may be linked to health problems. (For a list of artificial ingredients to avoid, see the "Think Simple" section on page 47.)

Keep in mind that since you're loading up on Mediterranean-style staples like fresh produce, whole grains, healthy fats, seafood, and beans most of the time, there's no reason to sweat the occasional high-quality steak or slice of homemade cake. When you enjoy them in moderation as part of an overall healthy diet, they aren't going to make you sick or cause your pants to end up too tight. What's more, indulging in these treats without the guilt keeps feelings of deprivation at bay—and can lead to a healthier, more relaxed relationship with food overall.

A DIFFERENT WAY OF LOOKING AT FOOD

We've talked all about how the Mediterranean diet is filled with fresh, mouthwatering foods that support your best health. But eating Mediterranean-style is about much more than just tossing a bunch of prescribed items into your cart and trying to force them into your eating habits. It's about learning to see food differently than what you might be used to.

Here at home, we tend to value convenience over freshness or flavor. (Frozen meals, anyone?) Busy schedules mean that speed and ease tend to win out over family dinners. And making healthy choices is often an all-or-nothing kind of game: If you're not being "good" by sticking to things like grilled chicken breast and salad, you're being "bad." Which usually leads to feeling guilty and over-eating. That's not how it is at most Mediterranean tables, though. There, fresh, whole foods are emphasized over processed ones—and *all* foods have a place in a healthy, well-rounded diet. Here are some of the overarching principles that most Mediterranean eaters abide by—and the reasons why they're worth incorporating into your routine.

FOOD COMES FROM NATURE

Step into a Mediterranean cook's kitchen, and you might spot ripe red tomatoes or a loaf of whole grain bread on the countertop. Chances are, there'll be a bouquet of leafy herbs and a jug of olive oil, too. Peek in the fridge, and you could see a tub of yogurt, a wedge of cheese, or a piece of fresh fish. Open up the cabinets, and find jars of whole grains, dried lentils or chickpeas, and maybe a bag of almonds or walnuts.

Here's what you probably won't see: Potato chips, sugary cereal, certain frozen meals, instant mac and cheese, store-bought cookies, or cupcakes. Above all, the Mediterranean diet emphasizes whole, minimally processed foods. Think, things that were pulled from the ground or plucked from a tree over ones that were spit out of a machine and packed into a box or bag. Unprocessed or minimally processed foods aren't just more flavorful; they are also loaded with nutrients that support your health, like phytonutrients and fiber, and are free of ingredients that do the opposite, like artificial additives or unhealthy fats. They can also help you lose weight: When Harvard researchers followed 120,000 healthy men and women for 20 years, they found that eating mostly whole, minimally processed foods—fruits and vegetables, whole grains, nuts, and yogurt—was associated with long-term weight loss, while eating mostly highly processed foods—potato chips, soda, and processed red meat—was associated with long-term weight gain.[51]

Does adopting a Mediterranean-style diet mean you can never buy any packaged foods again? Of course not. There are plenty of minimally processed foods or healthy food ingredients that usually *come* in a box or container, like plain yogurt or whole wheat pasta. What's more, convenience foods like jarred tomato sauce or prechopped frozen stir-fry veggies can help you get dinner on the table more efficiently. Just make sure to read the labels to look for foods with the least amount of added sugar and sodium. (For more help on shopping for packaged foods, see the "Think Simple" section on page 47.) And, of course, make sure that you love the way that they taste!

FLAVOR, FRESHNESS, AND QUALITY MATTER

At some point, you've probably choked down a mediocre sandwich from a fast-food chain or bitten into a hard, flavorless peach in the dead of winter. These lackluster experiences tend to be pretty disappointing, and they may have even driven you to raid the fridge or pantry later on in search of something more satisfying. *Even* if you aren't actually hungry.

In the Mediterranean, a meal is only as good as the ingredients that go into it—and a dish simply isn't worth eating if it's not delicious. That means seeking out quality foods that are fresh, in season, and free of questionable additives or preservatives. Not only are these types of foods better for you, they're just more enjoyable to eat. Take tomatoes, for instance. You don't need much more than a drizzle of olive oil and balsamic vinegar, plus a sprinkle of salt and pepper, to make a salad of juicy summer tomatoes taste truly mouthwatering. But no amount of dressing, croutons, cheese, or anything else will do much to improve their mealy winter counterparts. Why? Because imported or hothouse-grown winter tomatoes are never very good to begin with.

Of course, this sort of thinking doesn't just go for produce. No matter what the ingredient, the highest possible quality foods make for the tastiest, most satisfying meals and snacks. And often, that will allow you to eat less of the food or use a smaller amount in your cooking. It's easy to gobble up an entire sleeve of highly processed crackers made with white flour and sugar because they just don't have that much flavor or substance. But freshly baked whole grain bread dipped in extra-virgin olive oil? It's nutty, hearty, and chewy, so a piece or two is usually enough to hit the spot. It's a similar story with something like Parmesan cheese. You might be tempted to dump a big pile of the processed, canned stuff on top of your spaghetti marinara because adding just a spoonful might not add enough flavor. But shavings from a real wedge of Parmesan are rich and complex, and it only takes a little bit to take your pasta from good to spectacular.

So go ahead and let yourself be a little choosy. Seek out locally grown, in-season fruits and vegetables from the farmers' market. Splurge on the artisanal extra-virgin olive oil, cheese, or chocolate, and enjoy it in smaller quantities. Buy fresh whole grain bread from a local bakery instead of the squishy loaves that come in plastic bags. Head to a local fishmonger or butcher for the freshest fish, poultry, and meat. Your taste buds will notice the difference—and your body will reap the benefits.

■ *NOTHING* IS OFF-LIMITS

Bread. Potatoes. Pasta. Red wine. Rich desserts. And, of course, plenty of olive oil. Mediterranean meals incorporate all kinds of foods, including some that conventional dietary wisdom says you should avoid altogether. So how can an eating style that includes all of these foods actually be good for you?

It all comes down to moderation. Pasta tends to make a daily appearance on most Italian tables, but a serving might be just a few ounces, and it'll be eaten with plenty of fresh vegetables or a piece of fish—not exactly like the platter of fettuccine Alfredo you might get from your neighborhood joint with the red-checked tablecloths. Bread is served with most meals in Greece, not slathered with butter, but dipped in an infused olive oil or hummus. Throughout the Mediterranean, it's a similar story for many so-called forbidden foods, like rice, potatoes, dessert, or alcohol. A typical Mediterranean meal might include one glass of red wine, not four. It might occasionally end with a cookie or a slice of cake,

>>> **The Perks of Pleasure**

"A wise person does not simply choose the largest amount of food but the most pleasing food," wrote the ancient Greek philosopher Epicurus. Clearly, folks in the Mediterranean have been emphasizing food quality over food quantity for a long time! And sure, the idea sounds nice. But can giving yourself permission to have that side of pasta or square of dark chocolate *really* translate to healthier eating habits? The answer might be yes, suggests recent research. People who first see food as a source of pleasure in and of itself tend to eat smaller portions and score higher on measures of well-being compared to those who see pleasurable foods as the "enemy" to healthy eating, found a study published in the journal *Appetite*.[52] Permission to eat what you love? Granted.

but more often, dessert is fresh or poached fruit. And the portion size tends to be a few satisfying bites' worth, not enough to give you a stomachache.

In short, when you approach food the Mediterranean way, you don't have to say no to everything that's not kale or quinoa. By finding ways to balance out the fatty, heavier foods with healthier fare, keep portions in check, and treat yourself *sometimes* instead of every day, you can enjoy a little bit of everything. And you should! Because in the Mediterranean, food and pleasure really *do* go hand in hand.

FOOD SHOULD MAKE YOU FEEL GOOD

In the United States, it's common—almost normal—to have a love-hate relationship with your food. You might adore the taste of buttery shrimp scampi or sweet blueberry crisp with creamy vanilla ice cream, but after you eat them, you might feel a twinge of guilt, like you committed some kind of nutritional crime. On the other hand, having something like salad or fruit probably makes you feel virtuous. After finishing that meal, you might feel like you scored some major health-food points.

Things aren't so black and white when you follow the Mediterranean diet, which emphasizes that eating is a joyful, even sensual activity that's celebrated, not feared. That's because food isn't categorized as good or bad. Instead, food is just *food*. Sure, some things are intended to be eaten on a daily basis, and others are more of a once-in-a-while kind of thing, but whether it's an everyday Wild Greens Salad with Fresh Herbs (page 111) or an occasional Blueberry-Lemon Tea Cakes (page 77), it is always worth savoring.

How can a laid-back approach like this possibly help you eat healthfully? There are a few factors at play. First, we're talking about *real* foods—not highly processed, foodlike substances: sorry, neon cheesy puffs! By sticking to nourishment that comes from nature, you've already won half the battle. You don't have to worry as much about overdoing it on things like sugar, salt, or unhealthy fats, because whole foods—like the kind that make up the Mediterranean diet—naturally contain less of those ingredients.

Listening to your body plays a role, too. Eating a Mediterranean-style diet isn't just about honoring good food—it's also about honoring yourself. And chances are you'll be happy about your food choices if they make you feel good *physically*. That means eating moderate portions until you're satisfied, not stuffed. It also means saving richer, heavier fare like red meat or sugary desserts for special occasions instead of having them every day. After all, it's hard to feel lively and energized after polishing off a steak and an ice cream sundae, right?

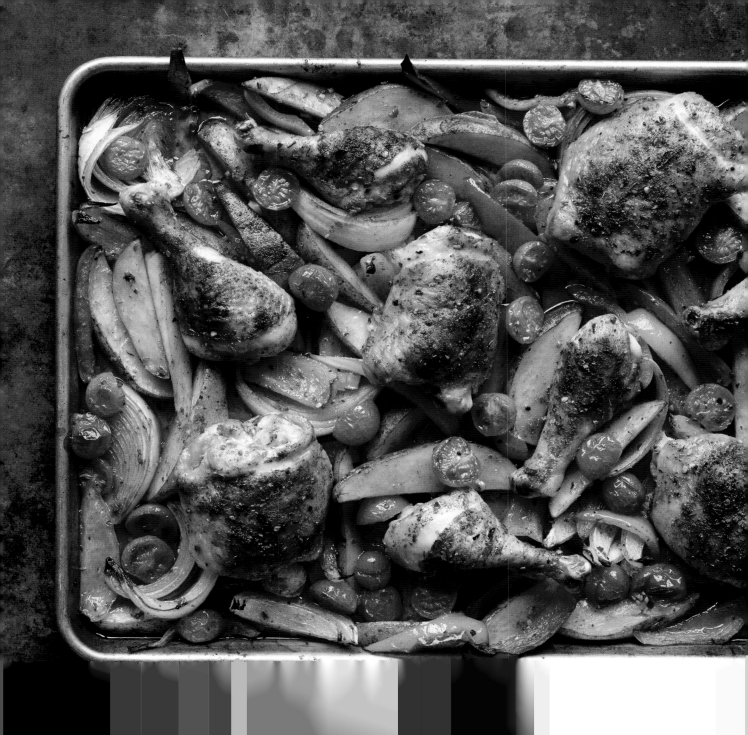

Chapter 2
Eating Mediterranean Anywhere

Whether you live on the sunny shores of Sicily, on the bustling streets of Madrid, or in Anytown, USA, incorporating a Mediterranean diet into your life is easier than you think. And you certainly don't have to live in the Mediterranean to *eat* like you do. Here's how you can give your diet a tasty Mediterranean-style makeover, plus a look at the staples you'll want to start keeping in your kitchen.

MAKING YOUR DIET MEDITERRANEAN

If you've ever eaten olive oil–roasted vegetables, a handful of nuts, or the occasional piece of broiled fish, good news: You're already enjoying a taste of the Mediterranean without realizing it. Following a Mediterranean-style diet is merely a matter of shifting many of the foods you already eat—fruits, vegetables, whole grains, healthy fats, and seafood—to the center of your plate. As you fill up on more of those, you'll naturally have less room for other, less healthy foods. You can still make space for the foods you enjoy, just in moderation. Remember there are no "good" or "bad" foods.

In other words, it's all about proportions. That's where these seven simple steps come in. Incorporate them into your eating habits, either one at a time over a gradual period to get the hang of things or all at once, if you'd like. Either way, they'll give you the tools you need to shift toward a Mediterranean style of eating and reap all of the incredible benefits that come with it. Here's how to get started.

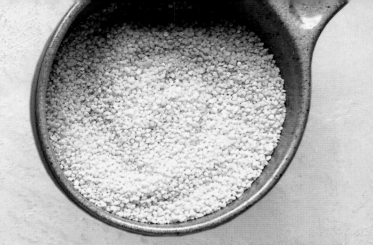

STEP 1: LET FRUITS AND VEGETABLES BE YOUR BASE

What's on today's menu? If you're like most Americans, the first thing that probably comes to mind is your protein. Here at home, meals often revolve around animal proteins like meat and poultry, with just a small helping of fruits or vegetables. Or none at all. Only 13 percent of Americans get the daily recommended 2 to 3 cups of vegetables, and only 24 percent get the recommended daily $1\frac{1}{2}$ to 2 cups of fruit.[1] For example, eggs and bacon with a wedge of melon for breakfast, a turkey or roast beef sandwich with a lettuce leaf and tomato slice for lunch, and a pork chop or some roast chicken with a few green beans or broccoli spears for dinner. Sound familiar?

In the Mediterranean, produce tends to play a starring role, sitting at the center of the plate instead of on the side. A typical Spanish or Italian breakfast, for instance, might be nothing more than fresh seasonal fruit with a piece of whole grain toast and some soft cheese. Various vegetable dishes—like simple chopped tomatoes, bell pepper, and cucumber, or smoky roasted carrots—paired with warm hummus and whole wheat pita make up the standard Israeli or Lebanese lunch. And whether it's enjoyed at the beginning or the end of the meal, most Mediterranean dinners aren't complete without a big green salad.

Indeed, Mediterranean eaters value fresh fruit and vegetables just as highly as we tend to prize those traditional, protein-based showstoppers. *Especially* when the produce is in season. After all, you can enjoy a piece of

25

salmon or some roast chicken almost anytime. But spring's tender asparagus, summer's candy-sweet corn, or fall's juicy figs may only be at their prime for a few short weeks. Not eating your fill would practically be a culinary crime!

Still, moving fruits and vegetables to the front might seem intimidating, especially if you're used to building most of your meals around meat. But with a little bit of practice, it's easy, especially once you start thinking Mediterranean-style. These tips can show you the way. (For more meal ideas, check out the plant-centric sample menus starting on page 276.)

• **GO WITH THE (SEASONAL) FLOW.** Trying to figure out a meal plan out of thin air can be tough. Instead, let the seasons be your guide. If the market is overflowing with artichokes or zucchini, for instance, there's a good bet that they're at their peak of deliciousness. So load up, and build your meals around these fresh ingredients.

• **DON'T OVERTHINK IT.** Most of the time, Mediterranean cooks treat produce simply, without a lot of fuss. As you begin adding more seasonal fruits and vegetables to your repertoire, you'll quickly find that they don't need much beyond a drizzle of olive oil, a squeeze of fresh citrus, or a dusting of chopped nuts or fresh herbs to taste incredible.

• **START WITH A PILE OF GREENS.** In many parts of the Mediterranean, it's not a meal without a heaping mound of green vegetables, like tender lettuces, sturdy kale or Swiss chard, or wild greens like dandelion greens. How about rethinking your usual mealtime ratios by having a large green salad and a smaller portion of protein? Or using raw or cooked greens as an edible bed for fish, chicken, or even pasta or rice dishes?

• **MAKE A MEAL OUT OF YOUR SIDES.** Take a cue from Spanish-style tapas or Middle Eastern meze platters, and make a meal out of several veggie-centric, appetizer-style dishes. Think Arnabit (*Roasted Cauliflower*) with Spicy Tahini Sauce (page 177), Warm Beets with Hazelnuts and Spiced Yogurt (page 182), and Halloumi, Watermelon, Tomato Kebabs with Basil Oil Drizzle (page 171). Sure, not having a main, meat-centric component might seem a little strange at first. But you'd be surprised by how satisfying a selection of small plates can be!

• **TREAT MEAT AS A FLAVOR-ENHANCER.** Rather than plunking a big piece of protein on your plate, use smaller portions in vegetable-based dishes. Try tossing a little bit of shredded chicken or turkey into a grain and vegetable pilaf. Or add a bit into stuffed vegetables along with plenty of whole grains, nuts, and herbs, like in the Stuffed Mini Peppers (page 179).

▌ STEP 2: GO FOR WHOLE GRAINS

If there's one thing the Mediterranean diet is not, it's low-carb. And yet Mediterranean-style eaters still manage to stay healthy and lean. How? Turns out, there's no big secret here. They simply enjoy their warm, chewy bread and pita, silky fresh pasta, and nutty pilafs in more moderate portions. And most of the time, they choose whole grains—or foods made from whole grains, like whole wheat pasta or bread.

Remember, unlike their refined counterparts, whole grains are rich in fiber. They fill you up faster and keep you fuller for longer, so you're likely to find yourself feeling surprisingly satisfied with smaller quantities. What's more, they promote stable blood sugar levels to deliver steady, even energy that lasts for hours—nixing the urge to nibble on sugary snacks in between meals. Can you say *any* of that about a plate of white pasta or a bowl of white rice? Probably not.

Best of all, the nutty flavor of whole grains is truly tasty—and adding more of them to

27

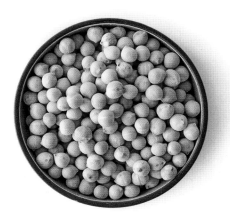

> ### ››› Is This Bread Whole Grain?
>
> Forget what you see on the front of the package. Wholesome as they might sound, terms like "whole wheat" and "multigrain" don't actually guarantee that a product is made with whole grains. Manufacturers often add a touch of whole grain flour to packaged breads, pitas, or wraps to make them look healthier. So how can you tell whether you're dealing with a real whole grain product or a cleverly disguised imposter? Just check the ingredients list. If a whole grain (like "whole wheat" or "whole oats") is listed as the first ingredient, you're probably in the clear. If you don't see the word "whole," the food in question is probably made mostly with refined flour. Also, keep in mind that whole grain/whole wheat bread should have at least 3 grams of fiber per slice.

your diet is simple. Often times, it's as easy as swapping out a refined grain for a whole one—like using whole wheat pasta or whole grain bread instead of plain white. But there are plenty of other creative ways that Mediterranean eaters get more whole grains in their diet, too. Like these:

• **SWAP CEREAL FOR PORRIDGE.** Cold cereals tend to be highly processed, and they're usually made with mostly refined grains, which explains why they never keep you full for more than an hour or two. Instead of a bowl of highly processed O's or flakes, try making a creamy breakfast porridge by simmering whole grains like whole wheat couscous or bulgur wheat in milk. Topped with fresh or dried fruit and a drizzle of honey, it's a seriously satisfying way to start your day.

(Try Fruit and Nut Breakfast Couscous on page 79.)

• **FORTIFY RECIPES WITH WHOLE GRAINS.** Their mild nuttiness fits in almost everywhere, so cook a batch at the beginning of the week, and add it to recipes all week long. Try stirring brown rice into soups, like in Harira (*Moroccan Chickpea and Lentil Soup*) on page 98, or make grain-enriched turkey or meatballs, like Lebanese-style Baked Turkey Kibbeh (page 188). You can also fold cooked grains into baked goods, muffins, or quick breads.

• **FIND NEW USES FOR BREAD.** When you eat Mediterranean, bread is not just for sandwiches. Toss crunchy toasted whole grain bread or pita points into a salad instead of the usual white croutons, like in Fattoush (*Leba-*

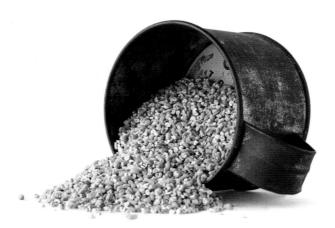

nese Pita Salad) on page 119 or Panzanella (*Tuscan Bread and Tomatoes Salad*) on page 126. Or use stale whole grain bread for thickening soups, like in Ribollita (*Tuscan Bean, Bread, and Vegetable Stew*) on page 100.

• **HALVE YOUR PASTA.** Add extra flavor and texture to pasta dishes by swapping half of your noodles for grains, like in Kushari (*Egyptian Rice, Lentils, and Ditalini*) on page 217, which is a mix of pasta and rice.

• **BAKE WITH WHOLE GRAIN FLOURS.** Whole wheat flour is one great option, but cornmeal, rye flour, or buckwheat flour are equally delicious. Try substituting half of the white flour for whole grain flour in your favorite cookies, cakes, and quick breads, or experiment with whole grain recipes like Blueberry-Lemon Tea Cakes (page 77), which are made with polenta.

▌ STEP 3: FLIP YOUR FATS

Without healthy fat, the Mediterranean diet would practically be unrecognizable. There wouldn't be any olive oil to drizzle over salads and cooked greens, add body to sauces like pesto or hummus, or create a crisp, caramelized crust on roasted vegetables or fish. There wouldn't be any nuts or seeds for stirring into yogurt or fresh ricotta cheese, folding into grain pilafs, or stuffing into vegetables. And

›› The One Fat to Always Avoid

Eating a Mediterranean diet means that you shouldn't fear fat, especially the monounsaturated kind. But partially hydrogenated oil, or trans fat, is pretty scary stuff. This synthetic, highly processed fat tends to show up in packaged foods, like margarines, baked goods, crackers, chips, coffee creamer, and fast food, where it helps improve texture and shelf life. The problem? Trans fats can raise levels of LDL, or "bad," cholesterol and increase the risk for heart disease, which is why the FDA has required that all food manufacturers stop using them by 2018. Until then, you can avoid trans fat by scanning a packaged food's ingredient list. If it includes partially hydrogenated oils, that means the food contains trans fat. That's true *even* if the nutrition label says 0 gram trans fat, since foods labeled as having 0 gram trans fat can still have up to 0.5 gram trans fat per serving.

there wouldn't be any plump, fruity olives for snacking.

Clearly, Mediterranean eaters aren't afraid of fat—and you shouldn't be, either. A splash of good-quality olive oil is sometimes all it takes to make a good dish feel positively rich and luxurious. And as we talked about in Chapter 1, fat-free and healthy simply don't go hand in hand. In fact, it's the opposite! The key, then, isn't cutting fat out of your diet. It's about choosing healthier sources of fat most of the time and eating foods that contain less-healthy sources of fat less often.

Not all fats are created equal. Emerging evidence suggests that the saturated fat found in things like butter may not be the very worst type of fat you can eat. (That award might go to trans fat. For more on why, see "The One Fat to Always Avoid" on page 29.) But monounsaturated fats from foods such as olive oil, avocados, and nuts actually do your body *good*—from helping you feel fuller longer, to lowering cholesterol and promoting heart health, to fighting oxidative stress that can lead to disease-causing inflammation. With so many amazing benefits, it makes sense to get your fill. Here's how folks in the Mediterranean do it and how you can, too.

• **MAKE OLIVE OIL YOUR GO-TO FOR COOKING.** Use regular or light olive oil for sautéing, roasting, grilling, and baking—it has a more neutral flavor, so it won't overpower your food. ("Light" olive oils are those with a lighter taste; they aren't lower in fat or calories.) Pick extra-virgin olive oil when you want its deep, grassy flavor to shine through (as well as for a bigger antioxidant boost). Think dressings, sauces, drizzling over finished dishes, or as a dip for bread.

• **CUT BACK ON THE BUTTER.** Butter isn't a common ingredient in most Mediterranean kitchens—most recipes don't call for it, and it's rarely spread on bread. It's fine once in a while in small quantities, but stick to using it only when the flavor is essential, like in special baked goods.

• **TRY NEW USES FOR NUTS AND SEEDS.** A handful of walnuts or almonds is always a smart snack choice, but you don't have to limit nuts and seeds to your midday nosh. You can also grind them in a food processor to use as a coating for chicken and fish instead of white bread crumbs, sub them for some of the flour in baked goods, puree them with olive oil and vinegar to add extra body to salad dressings, or add them to smoothies.

• **TAKE A LOOK AT YOUR CONDIMENTS.** Many store-bought mayonnaises are made with low-quality oils like soybean oil. If you like a spoonful of mayo on sandwiches or in spreads, opt for one made with extra-virgin olive oil instead. (Or if you'd like, make your own using the lemon-garlic aioli recipe on page 160.) Another option? Use other healthy fat sources to give sandwiches a flavor kick instead. Sliced avocado, olive tapenade, tahini, or hummus are all tasty choices.

• **GIVE YOUR MEAL A RICH FINISH.** Drizzling *more* olive oil on top of your food might seem a little scary. But Mediterranean eaters do it all the time—it's that final flourish that adds an extra hit of flavor and richness to finished dishes. (Ever wonder how the fish or veggies at that authentic Mediterranean-style restaurant taste so darn mouthwatering? Chances are *that's* why.) Of course, how much to add depends on your individual needs and nutritional goals. Fat is high in calories, so adding more to your meal might not make sense if you're trying to lose weight, but as a general rule of thumb, it's fine to drizzle your meal with a teaspoon, or approximately 50 calories' worth, of extra-virgin olive oil just before serving.

STEP 4: PICK LEANER PROTEINS

People living in the Mediterranean have long relied on lean sources of protein, like beans, fish, eggs, yogurt, and cheese. Though you might find red meat on the menu for very special occasions, things like spaghetti and meatballs or grilled lamb simply aren't a part of the daily diet for most Mediterranean eaters.

In the past, lean proteins were just cheaper to produce. Today, though, we also know how much better they are for your body. They're considerably lower in the saturated fat that can clog arteries and raise the risk for heart disease. But they're not just great because of what they *don't* have. Lean proteins like fish deliver hard-to-get nutrients like omega-3 fatty acids and vitamin D, while beans serve up their protein with a serious dose of fiber.

If pork or beef are staples in your kitchen, switching to leaner proteins most of the time might seem like a big step. But when you start thinking like a Mediterranean eater, you'll quickly see how easy it is to make delicious, versatile lean proteins the default for most of your meals.

• **EAT SEAFOOD AT LEAST TWICE A WEEK.** Seafood—especially fatty fish like salmon, tuna, trout, herring, and sardines—is low in saturated fat and rich in omega-3s, making fish and shellfish some of the healthiest protein sources you can eat. Aim to have two or three 3- to 4-ounce servings of seafood every week, and take advantage of the Mediterranean-style flavors and ingredients that can make fish and shellfish even more delicious. How about Roasted Branzino with Fennel, Lemon, and Olives (page 203) or Seared Scallops with Braised Dandelion Greens (page 200)?

• **GO BIG ON BEANS.** Several times a week, let beans and legumes be your meal's main protein source. They're especially satisfying in hearty soups like Cranberry Bean Minestrone (page 93) or main course salads like Spinach Salad with Pomegranate, Lentils, and Pistachios (page 112). But you can also pair them *with* smaller quantities of animal proteins, like in Chorizo, Shrimp, and Chickpea Stew (page 242). Fortifying a dish with beans makes it easy to cut back on the meat.

• **SWAP SWEET YOGURT FOR SAVORY.** Sure, low-fat yogurt and cottage cheese are always good with fruit. But they're wonderful in savory dishes, too. The tartness of low-fat yogurt pairs well with sweet vegetables, like in Warm Beets with Hazelnuts and Spiced Yogurt (page 182). Or try mixing cottage cheese with tomato, cucumber, fresh herbs, and olives to make Savory Cottage Cheese Breakfast Bowl (page 69) that's perfect with whole grain bread or pita.

• **SAY CHEESE.** Cheese doesn't show up at every single Mediterranean meal. But when it does, it adds a rich, savory flavor that's deliciously distinct. So opt for high-quality cheeses (no plastic-wrapped slices, please!) doled out in thoughtful doses—like in Arugula Salad with Grapes, Goat Cheese, and Za'atar Croutons (page 107) or Grilled Halloumi with Mixed Grilled Vegetables (page 127). (For more on the surprising health benefits of Halloumi, head to page 129.)

• **PICK POULTRY OVER RED MEAT.** Chicken and turkey tend to be lower in saturated fat and calories than red meat. Enjoy them a few times a week in dishes like Chicken and Olives with Couscous (page 241) or Grilled Rosemary-Lemon Turkey Cutlets (page 231), and save the beef or lamb for once or twice a month. Cured meats are often packed with unhealthy additives or preservatives, so choose fresh meat when possible. Just keep in mind that chicken can sometimes be a sodium bomb as a result of being saturated in a sodium solution. Read the label and find chicken that has no more than 70 milligrams per serving.

STEP 5: FIND FRESH SOURCES OF FLAVOR

A world without salt or sugar would be bland, indeed. Mediterranean eaters know that food falls flat without the right seasoning, and they have no qualms about using it to enhance a dish's flavor. But as with all things Mediterranean, the magic word is *moderation*. Having more than the recommended 2,300 milligrams of sodium per day can raise the risk for high blood pressure and stroke, while overdoing it on sugar can up the odds for obesity, diabetes, and heart disease.[2] (The American Heart Association recommends that women have fewer than 6 teaspoons, or 100 calories, of the sweet stuff daily; men, fewer than 9 teaspoons, or 150 calories.[3])

There's more, though. Think back to Chapter 1 when we talked about the value of picking out flavorful, high-quality ingredients—and how doing so can help you derive more enjoyment from your meals. Overseasoning can actually mask a food's inherent flavors, making it harder to pick up on all of those natural nuances and savor them fully. After all, a salt-laden dish just tastes, well, salty. And one with too much sugar tends be cloying.

Still, if you tend to lean heavily on the saltshaker or sugar bowl, cutting back can be tough. The good news is that Mediterranean-style food is intensely flavorful—thanks in no small part to the following small-but-mighty ingredients. Add more of them to your cooking, and you'll soon find that you need less of those other seasonings.

33

• **GARLIC.** These sweet, pungent cloves need no introduction. Next to olive oil, garlic might be the most commonly used flavoring in the Mediterranean. Simmer sliced garlic in olive oil before sautéing vegetables, rub chopped garlic on fish or poultry, roast whole heads and spread softened cloves on bread like butter, or combine it with olive oil and fresh herbs to make a marinade for fresh cheeses—like feta or mozzarella. Start your day off right with Garlicky Beans and Greens with Polenta (page 83)—just remember to brush your teeth (and tongue!) afterward!

• **FRESH AND DRIED HERBS.** From basil to parsley to thyme to rosemary to oregano to sage, Mediterranean-style cooking is chock-full of herbs. Not only are these flavor-boosters tasty; they're seriously good for you. Like veggies, both fresh *and* dried herbs are loaded with powerful phytonutrients. Use them in soups and broths, as a garnish on finished dishes, or stirred into sauces or dressings for a burst of fresh, savory flavor. Another idea? Try treating fresh basil, parsley, or dill like leafy greens, and toss them straight into a salad—like in Wild Greens Salad with Fresh Herbs (page 111) or Tabbouleh (page 186).

• **SPICES.** Just like herbs, ground spices, like cumin, coriander, turmeric, and smoked paprika, are highly concentrated sources of flavor and good-for-you antioxidants. What's more, spices that you might associate with sweet foods—like cinnamon, cloves, allspice, and nutmeg—aren't just for breakfast foods or desserts. They regularly show up in savory Mediterranean dishes, like in Crispy Spiced Chickpeas (page 152) and Grilled North African Spice-Kissed Sweet Potatoes (page 157).

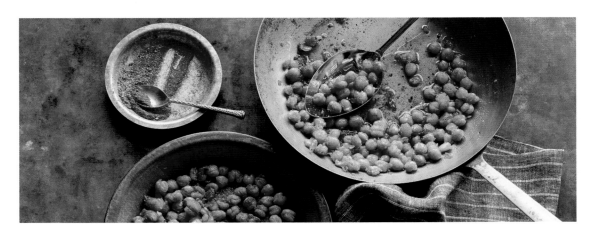

• **FRESH CITRUS.** When drizzled on at the end of cooking, fresh-squeezed lemon or orange adds a sharp, bright acidity that makes finished dishes pop. But don't just use the juice: Try folding finely grated citrus peel into yogurt or ricotta cheese or stirring it into salad dressings or soups.

• **HONEY.** This sticky syrup is a favorite in Mediterranean breakfasts and desserts—Loukoumades (*Honey Dumplings*) on page 253—and for good reason: Not only is honey more complex than refined white sugar, but it's also slightly sweeter. So you can get away with using a little bit less of it.

STEP 6: CHOOSE MINIMALLY PROCESSED SNACKS, DESSERTS, AND DRINKS

By now, we've talked a lot about how to Mediterranean*ize* your meals. But what about snacks and treats—where exactly do they fit in?

The good news is there's plenty of room for both. It's not unusual for folks to nibble on a little something in between lunch and dinner, which might not be served until 9:00 or 10:00 p.m. (The Spanish call this late-afternoon snack *la merienda*, while Italians call it *merenda*.) And, of course, it's impossible to talk about Mediterranean cuisine with-

out mention of the delicious desserts. Baklava, tiramisu, or flan, anyone? Still, Mediterranean eaters tend to approach between-meal bites and sweets a bit differently than we do here at home—and it's part of what helps them stay so healthy. To follow their lead, keep these tips in mind.

• **THINK SIMPLE FOR SNACKS.** This could mean sticking with snacks that are in their most natural, whole-food form—like fresh fruits and vegetables, nuts and seeds, or Crispy Spiced Chickpeas (page 152). Another option? Make a batch of a tapas-style snack that you can dip into throughout the week, like Cheese-Stuffed Dates on page 167, Muhammara (*Roasted Red Pepper and Walnut Dip*) on page 178, or Baba Ghanoush on page 154. Delicious options abound—just make it a point to pick fresh, wholesome snacks over highly processed ones.

• **END YOUR MEAL WITH FRUIT.** It's always worth indulging in homemade cookies or cakes on special occasions. But when it comes to everyday meals, most Mediterranean eaters enjoy fruit for a sweet ending. Eat what's in season—like berries in the spring and summer; apples, pears, or figs in the fall; and clementines or pomegranates in the winter—and make it feel special by serving it in a pretty bowl or platter, perhaps with some nuts or cheese (like the Fruit, Nut, and Cheese

35

Platters on page 258). Want to take things to the next level? Use fruit as a starting point for simple, seasonal desserts, like Grilled Apricots and Plums with Basil-Honey Yogurt (page 264), Spice-Poached Pears (page 262), or Almond-Peach Ice Pops (page 267).

• **SWAP SODA FOR UNSWEETENED BEVERAGES.** Aside from wine, the only other beverage you'll usually find on the Mediterranean table is water. Guzzling sugary drinks like soda is strongly linked to obesity, metabolic syndrome, and diabetes, and mounting evidence suggests that the artificial sweeteners in diet soda aren't much better.[4] Trade those plastic bottles for a pitcher of plain water (try adding sliced fruit or muddled herbs for extra flavor, if you'd like), sparkling water, or unsweetened iced tea.

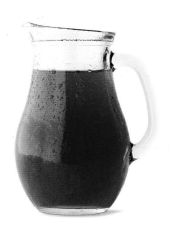

STEP 7: ENJOY ALCOHOL IN MODERATION

In wine-producing countries like Spain, Italy, and Greece, a meal simply isn't complete without a rich, fruity glass of vino. The right wine doesn't just make delicious food taste even better—savoring a glass of your favorite red or white encourages you to take your time, relish your meal, and enjoy the company of those around you. And unlike soda or other sugary drinks, it's actually good for you. We'll toast to that!

The one thing to keep in mind? Even though wine flows regularly at most Mediterranean tables, it doesn't flow *endlessly.* Save for special occasions and celebrations, most Mediterranean eaters enjoy one or two daily glasses of wine, max. And it's always sipped slowly with food, not guzzled on an empty stomach. These tips can help you take the same moderate approach.

• **PICK THE RIGHT DRINKS.** Make red wine your regular drink of choice. It's a top source of resveratrol, a polyphenol thought to promote heart health by protecting blood vessel linings and lowering levels of LDL, or "bad," cholesterol. Prefer white wine, beer, or spirits? You'll still reap some benefits since alcohol in general is thought to contribute to healthy blood vessel function and cholesterol levels.[5] Just save the cocktails for special

36

occasions—all that added sugar cancels out the alcohol's potential health benefits.

• **HAVE A GLASS OR TWO.** If you're a woman, have up to one drink per day; if you're a man, have up to two. (One drink is 5 ounces of wine, 12 ounces of beer, or 1.5 ounces of liquor.) Enjoying alcohol in moderate quantities is thought to boost your health. But experts *know* that drinking too much poses the risk for serious problems—including obesity, high blood pressure, liver disease, and certain cancers. If you have trouble with a middle-of-the-road approach to alcohol, it's best not to drink at all.

• **DRINK WITH YOUR DINNER (OR LUNCH).** In the Mediterranean, it's typical for wine to be enjoyed with a meal. Food helps slow the absorption of alcohol, and some findings suggest that compounds found in olive oil,[6] leafy green vegetables, beans, and whole grains[7] could even help counter alcohol's harmful effects, like blocking some carcinogenic compounds.

• **MAKE ALCOHOL OPTIONAL.** A Mediterranean-style diet doesn't *have* to include wine—or any alcohol at all, for that matter. If you choose not to drink or prefer to save drinks for once in a while, that's perfectly fine! Alcohol is far from essential. Though it may deliver some health advantages, the vast majority of the Mediterranean diet's benefits come from the food itself.

STOCKING A MEDITERRANEAN-STYLE PANTRY

Now that you know how to make your diet more Mediterranean, it's time to go food shopping. Don't worry, this isn't an authoritative list—and you don't need to buy all of these ingredients at once. Instead, use this as a guide for the types of foods that are worth keeping in your pantry and fridge. With them around, you'll always have the makings of a fresh, delicious Mediterranean-style meal.

▮ VEGETABLES AND FRUITS

It's easy to make fresh fruits and vegetables mainstays of your diet when you always have a variety in your kitchen. Pick one or two items from each of these categories, based on what's fresh, tasty, and in season at your local market.

• **LEAFY GREENS,** like romaine lettuce, kale, spinach, Swiss chard, and dandelion greens

• **COLORFUL VEGETABLES,** like cauliflower, cabbage, broccoli, asparagus, bell peppers, tomatoes, cucumber, eggplant, mushrooms, butternut squash, zucchini, and artichoke

• **AROMATIC VEGETABLES,** like onions, garlic, celery, fennel, and leeks

• **POTATOES,** including white and sweet potatoes

(continued on page 40)

37

››› Dining Out, Mediterranean-Style

No Mediterranean eater would deprive him- or herself the pleasure of the occasional restaurant meal. Dining out is a delicious treat, and restaurants are often the backdrops for memorable parties and gatherings. Who would ever want to give those things up?

At the same time, trying to make balanced, healthy choices when you're out to eat can sometimes be tricky. Restaurant meal portions are often two or three (or more!) times bigger than what you'd serve yourself at home. And because the food tends to be loaded with salt, sugar, and fat, putting down your fork isn't always easy—even once you feel full. At some point or another, we've all come home from a mouthwatering brunch or dinner nursing a serious food hangover. It's never fun.

The good news is that it's entirely possible to maintain your Mediterranean-style habits while dining out. And it doesn't matter what type of cuisine is being served, either. Whether you're at an authentic Italian trattoria, the local burger joint, or even a diner, you can still stick with the spirit of the Mediterranean diet by following these simple principles.

❖ **Arrive hungry, but not too hungry.** Sure, it's sometimes tempting to eat less throughout the day to "save up" for your restaurant splurge. But then, you run the risk of feeling ravenous when mealtime finally rolls around—which can set you up for overeating. Instead, stick to your normal, moderate portions throughout the day. If you're headed to the restaurant later than you'd normally eat, have a small snack (like a piece of fruit and some nuts) 2 or 3 hours before to hold you over. By the time you're seated at the table, you'll be hungry—but not so famished that you end up inhaling the entire breadbasket.

❖ **Pick a Mediterranean-style plate.** This doesn't mean that you have to order a dish with Mediterranean flavors (unless you want to, of course). What it does mean is that it's smart to look for options that have a Mediterranean-style balance of ingredients: Plenty of vegetables or fruit, whole grains instead of refined ones, lean protein over red or processed meat, and healthy fat. This might look like:

- Grilled or broiled fish with quinoa and vegetables roasted with olive oil
- Fajitas with corn tortillas and black beans, bell pepper, and red onion, topped with guacamole or shredded cheese

- Shrimp stir-fry with brown rice and broccoli with the sauce on the side for dipping
- Poached or scrambled eggs with whole wheat toast and fresh fruit
- A bowl of chicken and vegetable soup, a side salad with vinaigrette, and a whole grain roll

✣ **Make a meal out of appetizers.** You don't have to be at a Spanish restaurant to eat tapas-style. Instead of getting a full entrée, order a few smaller appetizers and veggie sides and share them with everyone at the table. You'll get to sample a little bit of everything, but you'll be less likely to go overboard on anything. Too much variety can cause us to overeat, so try to hit a balance here and make up a plate of what you plan to eat from the communal dishes and stick to that.

✣ **Clue in to keywords.** If the menu options still seem overwhelming, look for dishes that are baked, steamed, grilled, broiled, or poached, and skip those that are stuffed, crusted, or fried. They're lighter, and they're also less likely to be made with unhealthy fats commonly used by restaurants, like hydrogenated oils or margarine.

✣ **Keep your extras in check.** Plenty of Mediterranean meals feature wine, bread, and dessert—and there's no reason why you can't enjoy all three, too. But because restaurants here at home are more likely to be generous on the portions (automatic refill, anyone?), it's up to you to indulge without going overboard. Order one glass of wine, and sip it slowly throughout your meal. Have half a piece of bread, but pass on the butter. And if the desserts look *truly* delicious—not just so-so—order one with extra forks to share with the table.

✣ **Listen to your appetite.** Even a meal of fish, brown rice, and veggies can be too big. To avoid overeating, try checking in with your stomach halfway through. If you're full, put down your fork and have the rest of the food boxed up—you'll enjoy your meal more if you don't feel stuffed when you leave the table. Know you'll still have a hard time stopping? Split an entrée with one of your dining companions, or have your server bag up half of your meal before it even comes to the table. (For even more tips on mastering the Mediterranean art of moderation, head to the "Master Moderation" section on page 53.)

✣ **Take a walk.** Haven't you been meaning to try out that new restaurant less than a mile from your home? Now is your chance to walk there and back, adding some movement and extra quality time with friends or family into your day—both major components in the Mediterranean lifestyle.

- **FRESH FRUIT,** like apples, pears, berries, grapes, peaches, plums, pomegranates, cherries, oranges, and lemons
- **DRIED FRUIT,** like dates, figs, raisins, and dried apricots
- **FRESH HERBS,** like basil, parsley, dill, rosemary, thyme, mint, oregano, and sage
- **LOW-SODIUM JARRED OR CANNED VEGETABLES,** like artichoke hearts and roasted red peppers
- **OLIVES,** including kalamata and black

▮ WHOLE GRAINS AND BEANS

From bread for sopping up sauces and soups to grain porridges and pilafs to fast bean salads and dips, these humble staples are the workhorses of your pantry. Keep several of your favorites around, and you'll always be prepared to pull together a satisfying breakfast, lunch, or dinner.

- **WHOLE WHEAT BREAD OR PITA**
- **WHOLE WHEAT PASTA**
- **WHOLE GRAINS,** like brown rice, bulgur wheat, barley, polenta, and whole wheat couscous
- **ROLLED OATS**
- **WHOLE WHEAT FLOUR**
- **BPA-FREE, LOW- OR NO-SODIUM CANNED BEANS,** like chickpeas, white beans, and kidney beans (if you can't find low-sodium, rinse

the beans to remove about 40 percent of the sodium)
- **DRIED BEANS,** like lentils and split peas

▮ DAIRY AND EGGS

Look for pasture-raised products, when possible. Cows, goats, sheep, and chicken that mostly eat grass produce milk and eggs that contain higher levels of healthy fats compared to those who feed on grains and soybeans.

- **LOW-FAT MILK**
- **LOW-FAT PLAIN YOGURT,** either Greek or regular
- **LOW-FAT COTTAGE CHEESE**
- **FLAVORFUL HARD CHEESES,** like Parmesan and Grana Padano
- **SOFT CHEESES,** like ricotta, goat cheese, Halloumi, and feta
- **EGGS, CAGE-FREE AND ORGANIC WHEN POSSIBLE**

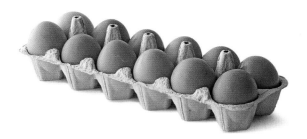

››› Should I Buy Organic?

It's a good idea to opt for organic when you can. Organic foods are produced closer to the way nature intended—without the use of synthetic pesticides, synthetic herbicides, and sewage sludge for plants, or antibiotics and hormones for animals. Research also suggests that some organic foods have more vitamins, minerals, and antioxidants,[8] and they might even taste better.[9] Organic foods also tend to be fresher since they don't contain preservatives to make them last longer.[10] Altogether, that could help you get more of the nutrients your body needs—and get the maximum amount of flavor from your food. At the same time, it's no secret that organic foods tend to be pricier—and they aren't always easy to find. So shop for organic when you can, but don't let that limit you. You'll always reap more benefits from conventional fruits and vegetables, whole grains, healthy fats, and lean proteins than by skipping something because it isn't organic.

▌ SEAFOOD AND POULTRY

For the most flavor, shop for fresh seafood or poultry the day you plan to cook it. Another option? Keep frozen or canned seafood and poultry on hand for easy meals anytime, minus the trip to the market.

• WILD-CAUGHT SALMON FILLETS, EITHER FRESH OR FROZEN

• SHRIMP, EITHER FRESH OR FROZEN

• WILD-CAUGHT OR US FARMED SHELLFISH, like mussels, clams, and scallops, either fresh or frozen

• BPA-FREE CANNED WILD-CAUGHT TUNA OR SALMON, PACKED IN OLIVE OIL

• BONELESS, SKINLESS CHICKEN OR TURKEY BREAST

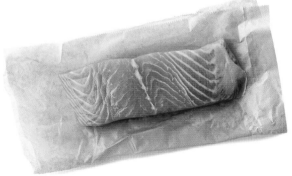

▌ OILS, NUTS, AND SEEDS

Look for cold-pressed or expeller-pressed oils—they're minimally processed, so they retain more nutrients and more flavor. If possible, store oils, nuts, and seeds in the refrigerator. Keeping them cold helps them stay fresher, longer.

- **EXTRA-VIRGIN, LIGHT, AND REGULAR OLIVE OIL**
- **RAW UNSALTED NUTS,** like walnuts, almonds, pine nuts, and pistachios
- **RAW UNSALTED SEEDS,** like flaxseed, sesame seeds, sunflower seeds, and pumpkin seeds
- **NUT AND SEED BUTTERS,** like almond butter and tahini (read the food labels and look for two ingredients in nut butters—the nut and salt—to avoid processed products)

>>> **Super Savings**

Good news: Eating Mediterranean is great for your wallet. Serving more produce, whole grains, and beans—and less meat—is an easy way to cut back on your food budget. In fact, eating a Mediterranean-style diet can save $750 in yearly grocery bills, according to findings published in the *Journal of Hunger & Environmental Nutrition*.[11]

42

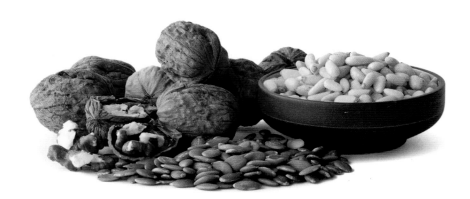

■ OTHER COOKING STAPLES

You'll only use a spoonful or two of most of these ingredients at once. But each one packs a distinct flavor punch, so it's smart to keep them stocked in your pantry.

- Honey
- Balsamic vinegar
- Boxed low-sodium chicken broth or vegetable broth
- BPA-free canned or jarred crushed tomatoes
- Tomato paste
- Dried herbs and spices
- Capers
- Anchovies

When you think about it, adopting a more Mediterranean diet is about making a few smart shifts—not embarking on a major overhaul. There's a good chance that you already enjoy plenty of the delicious, powerful foods that form the Mediterranean diet's base. It's simply a matter of bringing them to the center of your plate and having other foods less often. That's what makes following a Mediterranean diet so easy—and enjoyable.

At the same time, eating Mediterranean-style is about much more than just adding more whole grains, vegetables, or olive oil to your menu. It's a leisurely, more thoughtful approach to food that emphasizes the values of slowing down, eating as a family, and listening to your appetite to have the foods you love without overdoing it. Next, we'll talk more about why these things matter—and how you can make them happen for you.

43

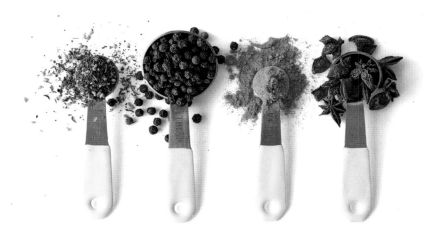

Chapter 3
Slowing Down to Savor

In the Mediterranean, leisurely meals tend to be the norm, beginning long before everyone heads to the table and ending well after the last bite is taken. Families might gather in the kitchen to share the cooking duties, working side by side to craft the meal.

When it's finally time to sit down, the courses start flowing: Often, there are appetizers or snacks. Then vegetables, followed by pasta or grains. Up next, there's the main course, and in places like Italy, there might even be a salad after that. Finally, there's dessert—maybe a cheese plate—along with plenty of sitting and chatting fueled by red wine and comfortable satiety that continues on long after the plates have been cleared and the sun goes down.

It's a little different than the way many of us eat in the United States: quickly polishing off a single plate and moving on from mealtime. Mediterranean eaters know that the key to eating well *and* eating for wellness is embracing high-quality foods and making them a central part of your life. What's more, they believe that celebrating great food and eating healthfully can—and do—go hand in hand. (Remember all of the Mediterranean diet's incredible benefits that we covered back in Chapter 1?)

The good news is that savoring your meals doesn't have to mean buying expensive ingredients or cooking for hours. It also doesn't mean that you need to spend the entire afternoon at a café or hosting weekly, multicourse dinners for your entire extended family.

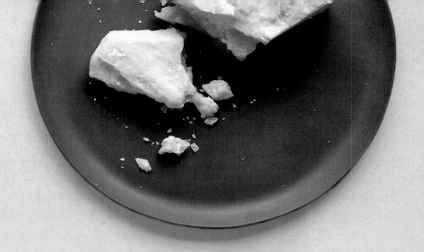

Though if you want to, you should go for it! You can adopt a Mediterranean-style attitude toward food that works with the lifestyle you already have. Here's how.

CHOOSE QUALITY OVER QUANTITY

Remember how most Mediterranean eaters believe food isn't worth eating unless it's truly delicious? Starting now, let that be your new mealtime mantra, too.

Maybe, at some point, you had a glass of wine that was so close to perfect you made the effort to sip it extra slowly so it would last as long as possible. Or you found yourself feeling genuinely satisfied after eating just half of that incredible plate of lobster ravioli or rich slice of chocolate fudge cake. We've all experienced those memorable dishes that seem to do so much more than just fill our bellies. *Those* are the kinds of meals that emphasize quality over quantity.

When you eat or drink something scrumptious, you refill your tank both physically and psychologically, and you're ready to move on to something else. Unlike the bland frozen entrée or the greasy drive-thru sandwich you might scarf down for the sake of convenience, high-quality foods can tamp down the temptation to eat past the point of satisfaction or root around in the kitchen for a snack an hour later. Over time, that can add up to pounds lost and health benefits gained.

That's not to say that your meals have to

be fancy, elaborate, or expensive. Far from it! Many of the most delectable Mediterranean recipes, including the ones you'll find starting in the next chapter, are simple dishes made from basic, unfussy ingredients. But the ingredients are always top quality—fresh, colorful, and nourishing—and *that's* what makes the final result taste great. Here's how to seek out the good stuff and make your meals worth the extra time.

▌ SHOP FRESH

It's not hard to find modern, one-stop-shop supermarkets throughout the Mediterranean just as you can in the United States. And yet, stopping daily—or almost daily—at the farmers' market, the bakery, the butcher, or the fishmonger remains part of the culture because the food is always fresher and tastier. Buying locally means that the food is in season, and it gives shoppers the opportunity to talk with growers and producers to get insider tips about what's delicious. Plus, heading to the market means that the ingredients for the day's meals are always at the peak of freshness. No slimy greens or overly ripe fruit here! All in all, food from local growers and specialized businesses is simply higher quality than the stuff at the grocery store, which loses flavor as well as nutrients after being flown in

from afar and sitting on the shelves for days or weeks.

Of course, our own culture functions differently, and, unfortunately, for most of us, getting to the market on a daily basis would be challenging. And even if you had the time to do so, making a meal almost exclusively out of local ingredients might still be tough—especially during the colder months. Even so, there are still plenty of cues you can take from the Mediterranean shopping playbook to find the freshest, most flavorful ingredients possible.

• **BUY LOCAL WHEN YOU CAN.** Frequent a nearby farmers' market, or consider purchasing a CSA (community supported agriculture) farm share. Both give you access to just-picked fruits and vegetables that are bursting with flavor. Even in the winter, you'll often find greenhouse-grown veggies, like kale or cauliflower, plus heartier produce, like winter squash, carrots, onions, apples, and pears.

• **STICK TO SEASONAL FOODS AT THE SUPERMARKET.** Many grocery stores now partner with nearby farms, so keep your eyes peeled for local and regional offerings, particularly in the produce section. Don't see any homegrown options? Try to still buy foods that are in season. Think strawberries and asparagus in the spring, tomatoes and peaches in the summer, pears and squash in the fall, and pomegranates and Brussels sprouts in the winter. They'll always have more flavor and better texture than their off-season counterparts.

• **THINK OUTSIDE THE VEGETABLE BOX.** Seeking out more locally grown produce isn't the only way to add fresh flavor to your diet. Chances are there are producers in your area selling locally raised eggs, poultry, and meat, as well as cheeses, yogurt, milk, bread, pickles, jams, and preserves. Seafood, too, if you live in a coastal region. It's just a matter of tracking them down. Check out localharvest.org to find out what's available in your area. You might be surprised! Make a trip to the farmers' market a fun family activity.

• **BREAK UP YOUR WEEKLY SHOPPING.** How about stopping at the farmers' market on your way home from work for salad ingredients or picking up fresh fish for tonight's dinner? When possible, make two or three weekly shopping trips instead of just one so nothing ends up sitting in your fridge for days (or weeks) before you get around to using it. Your resulting meals will be tastier for it—and you might find that your food waste goes down, too.

• **CONSIDER MEAL PLANNING.** If shopping multiple times a week is too much for you and your busy schedule and active family, you may consider carefully planning meals and keeping organized ahead of time so that you use your perishable foods first and frozen produce later in the week. Even taking a few hours on the weekend to make a hearty soup or cook a chicken can save you valuable time during the week and allow you and your whole family to eat healthier when all you need to do is reheat and eat.

▋ THINK SIMPLE

Eating a modern Mediterranean-style diet isn't about growing your own food and preparing everything from scratch. While fresh, minimally processed ingredients should make up the bulk of your diet, a few packaged foods can go a long way toward making life easier. The key is sticking with ones that are made from real ingredients (think, things your grandmother would recognize) and avoiding those that are highly processed, which often contain fake sweeteners, colorings, or preservatives. So before tossing that loaf of bread or bottle of salad dressing into your cart, always take a look at the ingredients list. If it's got any of the following sketchy additives, you may want to put it back on the shelf.

• **HIGH-FRUCTOSE CORN SYRUP (HFCS).** This highly processed version of fructose—the sugar that occurs naturally in fruit—often pops up in bread, yogurt, salad dressing, canned vegetables, and cereal. Eating too much of it can increase insulin resistance, raising the risk for diabetes and heart disease.

- **ASPARTAME, SUCRALOSE, ACESULFAME-K, AND OTHER ARTIFICIAL SWEETENERS.** These low- and no-calorie sweeteners are usually added to diet soda and sugar-free gum or desserts. They are linked to obesity and diabetes and could even have a negative impact on the good bacteria in your gut[1]—which is why many experts recommend avoiding them altogether.
- **TRANS FATS.** Partially hydrogenated oils, or trans fats, are a synthetic type of fat that's strongly linked to heart disease and diabetes.[2] Manufacturers are required to start phasing trans fat out of their products by 2018.[3] But until then, look for it in margarines, baked goods, crackers, chips, and fast food.
- **SODIUM NITRITE AND SODIUM NITRATE.** Avoid sodium nitrite, a synthetic preservative and possible carcinogen found in processed meats, like hot dogs, lunchmeats, bacon, and smoked fish. And limit your consumption of natural sodium nitrates, preservatives that are derived from celery and used in "uncured" meat products. They may be safer, but neither additive is good for you.[4]
- **BUTYLATED HYDROXYANISOLE (BHA) AND BUTYLATED HYDROXYTOLUENE (BHT).** Both

are petroleum-based preservatives that frequently make their way into potato chips, gum, cereal, frozen sausages, enriched rice,

---

››› Is This Food "Real"?

When you're stuck on whether a packaged food is truly nourishing and minimally processed, these guidelines can help.

1. Consider your choices. If you are debating frozen french fries, think about how simple it would be to make a baked potato. Or if you are reading the ingredients of an apple-flavored breakfast bar, think about how you could just eat an apple. Do you even need the packaged food in the first place?

2. Read the ingredients. Are they whole foods? Would it be easy to buy all (or most) of these ingredients at the grocery store? If so, those are good signs.

3. Check the sugar and salt. Yes, both are real foods—and it's perfectly fine to enjoy them in moderation. But packaged foods often have more than the body needs. Look for foods that do not have sugar listed as the first or second ingredient or contain multiple sources of sugar, and aim to keep sodium levels in packaged foods less than 800 milligrams per serving.

lard, and shortening. BHA is a likely human carcinogen, and BHT has been linked to cancer to a lesser degree.[5]

- **POTASSIUM BROMATE.** A flour bulking agent, potassium bromate is often used in bread and rolls, bagel chips, wraps, and bread crumbs as a dough strengthener. It could cause kidney or nervous system disorders and is a possible carcinogen.[6]
- **FOOD DYES LIKE BLUE #1 AND #2, RED #3 AND #40, YELLOW #5 (TARTRAZINE) AND #6.** Fake colors show up in everything from mac and cheese to candy to juices to maraschino cherries and more.

But you don't want (or *need*) them in your food: They're petroleum-based, and several have been linked to hyperactivity in kids and cancer in lab animals.[7]

- **CARAMEL COLOR.** Soda, beer, brown bread, chocolate, baked goods, and ice cream are where you'll usually find this common food coloring. It's processed with ammonia, which leads to the creation of the potentially carcinogenic compound 4-methylimidazole.[8]
- **MONOSODIUM GLUTAMATE (MSG).** A flavor enhancer, MSG is often found in potato chips and snacks, cookies, seasonings, canned soups, frozen meals, lunchmeats, and some Chinese food. It triggers migraines in some people[9] and has a highly addictive flavor that makes it hard to stop eating.

MAKE YOUR MEALS AN EXPERIENCE

Sit down at a table in Morocco or Malta, and the food you eat will almost certainly be different than what you'd have in Sicily or the south of France. But no matter where you are in the Mediterranean or what's on the table, there's one thing you'll almost always find: a communal, warm atmosphere.

In the Mediterranean, *what* you eat is pretty darn important. But *how* you eat matters just as much, if not more. Meals are events, and they're meant to be enjoyed at a relaxed pace, in the company of others, at the table. (Or in another environment with a great vibe and minimal distractions, like in a park or on a beach.) And unlike a sandwich or salad eaten alone in the car or while watching TV, meals go beyond just filling our stomachs.

Whether it's a romantic, candlelit dinner for two or a boisterous family brunch, meals satisfy our need to gather in a comforting space and connect with others. They also give us a much-needed break from the looming busyness that threatens to leave us worn out and exhausted. In other words, they're a delicious opportunity to slow down and come together with the people you care about. And that's something you can do whether

49

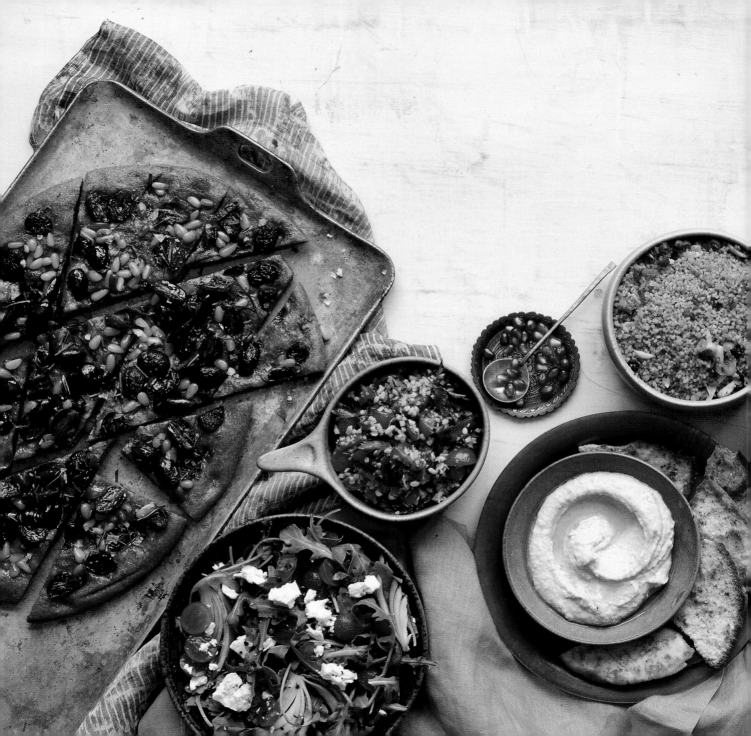

you live in the Mediterranean or not. Here's how to make them happen more often.

▎SHARE YOUR FOOD

Think about some of the best, most memorable meals you've eaten. Sure, the food probably tasted incredible. But chances are the people around you were what really made the magic. Maybe both you and your best friend groaned at the same time you bit into your meals, or you found yourself in an engrossing conversation over a dinner that went on for hours. Perhaps your favorite song came on just as you were putting a fork to your lips, and your spouse grabbed you so you could share a dance. Whatever happened, things *clicked*, and you made a memory worth treasuring. The food might have been part of it, but it certainly wasn't all of it.

People in the Mediterranean know that meals are always more meaningful when they're shared with family or friends. The food itself is always important—with so much emphasis on high-quality ingredients, how could it not be? But it's the people you're sharing the meal with that turn it into something special. Of course, getting everyone together—and keeping them at the table for more than a few minutes—isn't always easy! These real-life tips can help.

• **MAKE COOKING PART OF THE FUN.** Treating food prep as part of the festivities instead of a chore to rush through sets a relaxing tone for your meal. And you don't have to do it alone. Invite your friends or family members to help out with easy, low-stress tasks like washing salad greens or stirring the soup pot. Start cooking a little bit earlier, and take your time so you don't feel rushed. Or set out some light snacks for everyone to enjoy while you get the meal together, like raw vegetables with hummus or olive tapenade.

• **SCHEDULE MORE FAMILY MEALS.** They might not be possible every single night or morning, but it's worth getting the whole gang around the table as often as you can. Remember, conversation and connection are what separates a *meal* from simply *eating*—even if the only thing on the table is a basic salad or a pot of soup. Shared family meals have been shown to foster healthier eating habits in kids, too.

• **START A NEW TRADITION.** It could be making homemade pizza on Friday night or having the kids cook breakfast on Saturday morning. The menu itself isn't that important. It's really about forming family rituals that bring people together—and that hold steady even when life gets chaotic.

• **LET YOUR MEAL UNFOLD.** A typical Mediterranean meal might last 2 hours or more. You

51

> ### ›› Everybody In!
>
> Cooking with your child is an opportunity to share kitchen know-how, pass down family recipes (like the secret to Grandma's sauce), and get her excited about eating something other than the usual chicken fingers. And there are plenty of ways for kids of all ages to get involved.
>
> ❖ **Toddlers** might be too young to help with food prep, but they can still get in on the fun and feel like they're contributing. Give them an empty bowl or pot and some wooden spoons so they can pretend to mix and stir.
>
> ❖ **Preschoolers** can tackle basic hands-on tasks like tearing greens, stirring batter, or tossing salad.
>
> ❖ **School-age kids** can practice math skills by weighing and measuring ingredients. Some may also be mature enough to cut soft foods—like cheese or tomatoes—with a dull knife.
>
> ❖ **Tweens and teens** are old enough to tackle tasks like chopping and sautéing. With supervision, of course!

might not have *that* much time, but try to stretch your meal to a full half-hour. You'll quickly find that pacing yourself is more pleasurable than scarfing down your food at breakneck speed. Plus, eating at a slower speed gives your brain more time to get the signal that your stomach is full, helping you eat less overall.

• **HANG OUT FOR A WHILE.** Nothing kills the magic of a great meal more than jumping up to do the dishes the minute everyone puts down their forks. So sit a while longer and let the conversation continue to flow. In Spain, they call this *sobremesa*—and no meal is complete without it.

▌ TAKE YOUR MEAL UP A NOTCH

You might already pull out all the stops for events like birthdays or holidays, but *every* meal is worth celebrating in its own small way. After all, there's just something about setting the table and sitting down to eat that makes food taste better, right? So find ways to do it as often as you can. Sure, it might mean a few more minutes of work before you can dive in and start eating. But that little bit of extra effort is a big part of what makes your breakfast, lunch, or dinner feel special—and more like a welcome pause from the day instead of an indistinguishable part of the craziness.

Best of all, setting the mood doesn't have to involve a pristine white tablecloth or fancy flowers. Just like with Mediterranean-style cooking, simpler is almost always better. And these meal-elevating steps are simple enough to take every day.

• **SET THE TABLE.** You've got the dishes, glasses, and utensils—and maybe even some cloth napkins. So put them to work! Setting the table sends the unmistakable signal that it's time to sit down and eat, not wander off to the TV and eat or scroll through your phone and eat. What's more, research suggests that the heft of real plates and bowls can actually make your food feel more satisfying than flimsy paper or plastic ones.[10]

• **ADD SOME DÉCOR.** Want proof that all you need is a little extra something to make an everyday meal suddenly feel *nice*? Try putting a few freshly plucked wildflowers in a vase or filling a pretty bowl with fresh oranges or lemons, and see the difference it makes.

• **PAY ATTENTION TO PRESENTATION.** Make your food look pretty on the plate by adding a little garnish, or pile it onto good platters before bringing it to the table to eat family-style.

• **LOWER THE LIGHTS.** Soft lighting makes *any* atmosphere feel warm and inviting. So turn down the dimmer, light a few candles, or string a strand of twinkle bulbs around the eating area.

• **TURN UP THE TUNES.** Music is just another way to imbue your meal with ambiance. And unlike the distracting chatter from the TV, it won't kill the conversation by stealing everyone's attention. Make a dinnertime playlist with all your favorites, or stream a curated, commercial-free mix of jazz or classical songs.

MASTER MODERATION

When it comes to a Mediterranean-style diet, the term *moderation* gets tossed around a lot. It's key for enjoying things like bread, cheese, or dessert—and feeling good about it. Moderation also helps you get the biggest benefit from healthy foods or drinks, since in some cases, you really *can* have too much of a good thing. For instance, drinking too much alcohol can raise the risk for high blood pressure and some cancers, while overdoing it on calorie-dense olive oil or nuts could make it harder to lose weight.

Problem is, moderation can be a tough concept to grasp. Even the definition—avoiding extremes or excesses—is a little vague, and different people tend to interpret it in different ways. For some, enjoying chocolate in moderation might mean having a small square each

53

night after dinner. For others, it might mean indulging in a fudgy brownie once or twice a month, but not more than that.

Regularly being surrounded by supersized servings doesn't help, either. They can distort your perception of what healthy portions look like, so you end up piling too much food on your plate.

In the Mediterranean, concepts like moderation and portion control are simply part of

>>> **Communal Meals = Healthy Meals**

Eating as a family is more than just a chance to ask about how school was today. It's also one of the best times to model good eating habits, which can help get kids on the road to making healthy choices for life. Children who regularly eat with their families consume more wholesome foods, like fruits and vegetables, grains, and dairy, and fewer sugary sodas or fried foods, according to one *Advances in Nutrition* review.[11] That can help reduce the risk for obesity and up the odds that kids continue making healthy choices on their own as adolescents.

Of course, getting everyone together isn't always easy. There's always dance class and soccer practice getting in the way! But with a little bit of persistence, it's possible to make family meals a priority. Here are a few ways to have them more often—and make the most of them every time.

✣ **Set a weekly minimum.** If eating together every night isn't realistic, strive for at least three family meals per week. That's still often enough to have a meaningful impact on your child, experts say.[12]

✣ **Mark your calendar.** Treat family dinners just like soccer practice or doctor appointments. They'll be less likely to get cancelled or overlooked if they're on the schedule.

✣ **Go beyond the dinner table.** If evenings tend to be chaotic, have breakfast together instead. As long as everyone is eating together, you'll reap the same benefits at 7:00 a.m. as you would at 7:00 p.m. (For more tips on making sit-down breakfasts a reality, see page 66.)

✣ **Be in the moment.** Turn off the TV, put away the phones, and focus on spending time with each other. Put devices in another room; even the beep of a notification or text from the phone in your pocket can disrupt the family flow. Ask your child about his day at school, his friends, or his upcoming plans—and share what's happening in your life, too.

the culture. Indulgent foods are saved for special occasions, and it's considered unusual to scoop yourself a second serving of pasta or take a second slice of cake. That isn't always the case here at home, but here's the upside: As you adopt a Mediterranean diet, you might find that your approach to food starts to naturally shift and become more moderate. For instance, adding more healthy fats and whole grains to your meals could mean that you start to fill up faster, leaving you less interested in going back for seconds. And when you know that it's perfectly okay to enjoy a side of whole wheat pasta or a wedge of fruit tart, you might come to find that you don't actually want those things every single day. That might sound hard to believe now, but eating Mediterranean-style is not built on the principles of self-denial and sacrifice other diets are built on.

Even so, having *some* specifics about what moderation is—and isn't—can be helpful, especially when you first start eating more Mediterranean-style. That's where these guidelines come in.

GET REAL ABOUT PORTION SIZES

Whether at home or in a restaurant, portions in the Mediterranean tend to be significantly

>>> **Step Outside**

People have been eating outside since, well, the beginning of time. But you might argue that those living in the Mediterranean perfected the art of outdoor dining. After all, *alfresco* is a borrowed Italian term that means "in the cool air." (Though, these days, Italians are more likely to call outdoor dining *fuori* or *all'aperto*, meaning "out" or "open air." The Spanish have a similar term, *al aire libre*.) No matter what you call it, make the effort to enjoy more of your meals outside during the warmer months. From chirping crickets to glowing sunsets, Mother Nature always manages to create the kind of atmosphere that makes you want to linger just a little bit longer.

smaller than what you usually find in the United States. As a result, most Mediterranean eaters are simply used to eating less of, well, everything. An individual serving of pasta is usually served on what most of us would consider an appetizer plate, not piled high on a platter. Wine is poured into small glasses, not goblets. And a piece of fish, chicken, or meat might take up a quarter of the dinner plate instead of the entire thing.

The good news is that by paying close attention, it's easy to keep your portions balanced and eat more moderately. And you don't have to turn to rigid methods like weighing or measuring every morsel of your food. (That would be very un-Mediterranean, don't you think?) Make these simple serving checks a part of your regular routine, and over time, they'll start to feel like second nature.

• **KEEP FRESH FOOD OUT—AND PUT SNACKS AWAY.** You're more likely to reach for the foods you spot first, so keep fresh fruit out in a bowl on the counter where it's easily visible. Store sweets and treats in the cupboard or in the freezer so you're not tempted to grab a handful whenever you walk into the kitchen.

• **DOWNSIZE YOUR PLATES, BOWLS, AND GLASSES.** On average, we eat more than 90 percent of whatever is in front of us.[13] By simply using a smaller plate, bowl, or glass, you'll serve yourself less—and effortlessly end up eating less as a result.

• **MEASURE YOUR FATS.** It's easy to go overboard when you pour olive oil straight from the bottle. So when a recipe calls for it, grab your measuring spoon and use the exact quantity called for. You'll have enough to complement your dish, but it won't be more than you need.

• **PLATE YOUR FOOD IN THE KITCHEN.** Yes, family-style platters look bountiful on the table, but they can also make it extra easy to help yourself to more food—even when you are not actually that hungry. If you find that you're often tempted to take another bite or spoonful, try serving your meals already plated instead. You can still get up and take more from the kitchen if you really want to—after you have given yourself time to let the fullness settle in. But you'll think twice before you do it.

• **MAKE HALF OF YOUR MEAL VEGETABLES.** Chances are eating a Mediterranean-style diet means you're already bumping up your veggie consumption. So let them fill a full half of your plate. With vegetables taking up so much real estate, you'll automatically have less space for foods that are easier to eat too much of—such as pasta or grains and proteins like fish, poultry, or meat.

• **PORTION OUT YOUR SNACKS.** Put nuts in a small bowl (or plastic bag, if you are packing them to enjoy later) instead of noshing straight from the container. Cut a few slivers of cheese for yourself instead of setting out a big chunk. Portioning your snacks is a simple way to avoid accidentally overdoing it. And when you know exactly how much you have, you'll be more likely to eat slower and savor your food.

DEFINE SPECIAL OCCASIONS

Part of eating a Mediterranean diet means that every meal is worth celebrating. Whether it's a simple bowl of lentil soup or a multi-course holiday feast, it's always worth taking the time to set the table, sit down, and eat at a relaxed pace that allows you to really enjoy each bite, preferably, with family or friends beside you. But celebrating doesn't necessarily mean indulging. After all, a treat isn't a treat if you have it all the time, right?

The Mediterranean region is known for its lavish multicourse feasts. You know, the kind where countless friends and family members are gathered at a long table and large platters are piled high with rich, mouthwatering food. But, obviously, these sorts of fantastic fetes don't happen every day. Could you imagine how much work that would be? Instead, in addition to major holidays like Easter and Christmas, countries like Greece have feast days often centered on holy saints or other significant events. And during *il Carnevale*, the period between the Epiphany and Lent, Italians host celebrations marked by balls, parades, music, and, of course, plenty of traditional treats.

The special occasions that matter to you and your family might, of course, be different. Perhaps no birthday is complete without Aunt Sally's famous chocolate layer cake. Or you always make pot roast and pie when your far-away family members come to visit. No matter what, special treats can always be a part of significant events, especially when they play a role in honoring your family's traditions or values.

The key to eating moderately, then, is figuring out which occasions count as special ones that warrant indulging—and which ones don't. A weekly trip to the movies might not be a big enough deal to justify candy and buttery popcorn—especially because the snacks aren't even all that tasty. After all, does anyone really like the taste of artificial butter? But it might be worth treating yourself to a top-quality steak at a celebratory dinner or a gooey chocolate chip cookie from an incredible bakery while you're on vacation. In short, it's all about weighing your options and deciding what's important and what you can probably live without. There's no right or wrong answer, as long as *you* feel good about your choices.

EAT MINDFULLY

Mindful eating is often a trending topic these days, but it isn't exactly a new concept. Eating mindfully simply requires listening to your

57

appetite to decide what to eat and paying attention to your food while you eat it—two practices that are deeply ingrained in Mediterranean culture. Eating mindfully is closely connected to eating moderately: When you eat according to what makes you feel best and give your meals the focus they deserve, you're less likely to overdo it and feel uncomfortably full.

That can add up to big benefits. Findings show that people who practice mindfulness—including with their meals—are 34 percent less likely to be obese compared to those who rush around without paying attention.[14] They are also less likely to develop heart disease,[15] have healthier blood sugar regulation, and have a lower risk for diabetes.[16] Multitasking during a meal also steals some of your brain's attention, leaving you less able to experience the flavors fully, suggests one recent study.[17] So in addition to seriously improving your health, the simple act of mindfulness can actually help you enjoy your food more.

By now, it's probably no surprise that most Mediterranean eaters tend to eat mindfully by default. And many of the mealtime rituals we've talked about so far in this chapter, like sitting down at the table and letting your meal unfold slowly, can help you do exactly that. But there are other, more subtle ways

that Mediterranean eaters practice mindfulness to reap the maximum pleasure from their meals. Here's how you can, too.

▌ SLOW DOWN

Treat mealtime as an opportunity to relax and recharge, rather than as a race to clean your plate. Noshing at a more leisurely pace allows you to truly enjoy your food by taking notice of the flavors, aromas, and textures. What's more, eating slower gives your brain ample time to pick up on your stomach's fullness signals, so you're less likely to overeat. If you're used to speed-eating, try employing tactics that can help you pace yourself: Put down your fork in between bites, take frequent sips of your water or wine, and let yourself pause when you get engrossed in the conversation. Your food isn't going anywhere!

▌ DITCH THE DISTRACTIONS

Think back to the last time you scarfed down breakfast in the car, gobbled up lunch while answering e-mails, or munched on dinner as you stared at the TV screen. For most of us, we've done at least one of those things—if not all three—pretty recently. It might even be something you do every day as part of your routine. Are the details of the meal itself murky? Well, that makes perfect sense.

It's easy to shovel forkfuls into your mouth while you're doing something else. But you probably won't pay much attention to what—or how much—you're actually eating. When you're surrounded by distractions, it's harder to focus on the experience of enjoying your food, not to mention notice when you're starting to feel full. Together, that adds up to a bland eating experience where you leave the table (or the couch or desk) uncomfortably stuffed. That doesn't sound very pleasurable, does it?

For most Mediterranean eaters, food isn't something to squeeze in while you tackle other items on your to-do list or something to keep your hands and mouth occupied while watching TV or scrolling through social media. Meals are an event unto themselves—and often, they're *the* most important parts of the day. In many Mediterranean countries, lunch is an hours-long event where work comes to a grinding halt. And dinner is an opportunity to relax and reconnect with family after a busy day. Multitasking simply isn't part of the equation.

If you're making the effort to share more meals around the table, you may already be dining with fewer distractions. But eating with family and friends doesn't guarantee that attention juggling won't be a part of the meal. After all, we've all left the TV blaring in the background during dinner or eaten in near silence while everyone taps away at their phones. So take action! When eating at home, make the effort to turn off the TV and encourage your dining companions to put their phones in another room, preferably on silent mode. Without all that interference, you'll talk more and connect more deeply. And most likely, you'll find yourself eating a lot less, too.

As for work? You might not be able to steal away for an hours-long lunch, as is often customary in Italy, Spain, or southern France. But you can take some time to head outside to a bench, public park, or even to the communal break room instead of eating at your desk. Leave your phone behind, too, if you can. Even if it's just 15 or 20 minutes, you'll come back feeling calmer and more refreshed. And after enjoying your meal fully, you just might find yourself less interested in raiding the snack drawer or hitting the vending machine midafternoon. (For more ideas on how to slow down at lunchtime, see page 88.)

EAT WHAT YOU *REALLY* WANT

Have you ever eaten a salad because you felt like you "should" have it or scarfed down an entire sleeve of cookies because you had already "blown it" for the day? Chances are the answer is yes. At some point or another, we've all eaten something for reasons that have nothing to do with hunger or appetite. Maybe fear of gaining weight pressured you into picking the lower-calorie option. Or you felt the need to eat as many treats as possible before getting back on the healthy-eating wagon in the morning.

It's no secret that there are fewer heavy adults in the Mediterranean than in the United States. At the same time, most Mediterranean eaters don't worry nearly as much about whether they're eating "clean" or "healthy." They just eat! They eat when they're hungry, opting for the foods that

---

⋙ Delicious Habits

Mealtime rituals don't just help bring people together. They can actually make food taste better, according to findings published in the journal *Psychological Science.*[18] Food-centric traditions can make you feel more involved with your meal, so you enjoy it more fully. It's sort of like how kids are more excited to try foods they helped prepare; being hands-on is just more fun! And these practices don't have to be elaborate to be effective. Here are five simple ones worth trying.

❖ **Plan your weekly menu.** On the weekend, sit down as a family and figure out what dinner will be for the upcoming week. Menu-planning helps kids learn how to build healthy meals and makes weeknight dinners feel less harried. Plus, everyone can look forward to their favorites.

❖ **Give thanks.** Before digging in, take a minute to express gratitude for the food you're about to eat—and the people you're sharing it with.

❖ **Pick a playlist.** Make it a nightly habit to play music during the dinner hour. Assign each family member a night of the week to create a playlist for ahead of time.

❖ **Share your highlights.** Go around the table and invite your family to talk about the best thing that happened to them that day.

❖ **Clean up as a crew.** It's less of a chore when everyone pitches in. Turn it into a challenge by seeing how quickly you can get the table cleared and the counters sparkling again.

sound the most appealing, rather than weighing the pros and cons about fat grams or carbs. And they stop when they're satisfied, not feeling worried or guilty about how the meal might have impacted their caloric budget. Most likely, calories are hardly on their radar at all.

The takeaway here isn't that you should feast on pizza or creamy fettuccine every day and expect to lose weight or improve your health. Because you certainly wouldn't. Instead, it's this: It's worth paying more attention to your inner cues than to all of the outer ones. What are you really in the mood

››› Moving, Mediterranean-Style

We all know that regular exercise is an important part of losing weight and improving overall health. But that doesn't mean that you need to slog it out for hours on a treadmill. Expensive gym memberships and grueling boot camp classes simply aren't a part of traditional Mediterranean culture. And for good reason: They don't have to be!

From foraging for wild greens on the Greek islands to walking through bustling cities like Barcelona or Rome, Mediterranean lifestyles tend to be naturally active, so there's less of a need for formal exercise. And you can take a similar approach. By finding ways to build more movement into your day, you'll up your activity level without having to tack a trip to the gym onto your to-do list.

✣ **Make a 1-mile rule.** If a trip is a mile or shorter, consider walking or biking instead of driving. Over the course of 4 months, doing this alone could add up to a 3-pound weight loss, suggests one University of Michigan study.[19]

✣ **Find active activities.** Chances are you spend most of your weekdays seated at a desk. So consider taking up a hobby that keeps you on your feet in your free time, like dancing or tennis.

✣ **Get in the garden.** Growing your own fruits, vegetables, or herbs doesn't just give you access to the freshest produce possible. It helps you move more, too.

✣ **Take a walk just because.** In some Italian cities, it's common for families to take a predinner stroll, called *la passeggiata*, to unwind, socialize, and simply show off how great your outfit is. Give it a try—even if you'd rather just wear your comfiest sweats.

✣ **Meet up with friends.** Do something fun with friends instead of getting a meal or cocktails to mix things up. Maybe organize a kickball game or just take a walk in the park together.

for today? Would something warm and hearty like roast chicken with potatoes and vegetables hit the spot? Or do you need something lighter, like a green salad with a side of humus and whole wheat pita? Would the sweetness of a fresh piece of fruit be enough to satisfy you? Or is it a day where only a buttery cookie will do? If you take the time to check in with your appetite, it will give you the answer.

And whatever you decide is okay! Keep in mind, when you stick to a Mediterranean-style diet filled with fresh produce, lean proteins, whole grains, and healthy fats, you'll reap significant benefits from virtually any foods you choose. Since your cupboards are filled with wholesome foods to begin with, there's no need to worry about making the "best" choice. They're all great! At the same time, your diet will automatically have less room for sugary snacks, red or processed meat, or other items that could put you at higher risk for health problems if you have them too often. So when you *do* decide to treat yourself, you can feel good about it, not guilty.

Fresh, wholesome ingredients define the flavors of the Mediterranean diet, and they can go a long way toward protecting—or even improving—your health. But it's the cultural values surrounding the food that makes this style of eating truly nourishing. As you start incorporating more Mediterranean-style meals into your daily menu, think about how you can enjoy more of those meals in a relaxed setting with the people you care about. Just as important, check in with your appetite to determine the foods and quantities that would satisfy you the most. With an approach to food this enjoyable, it won't be long before these considerations start to become second nature.

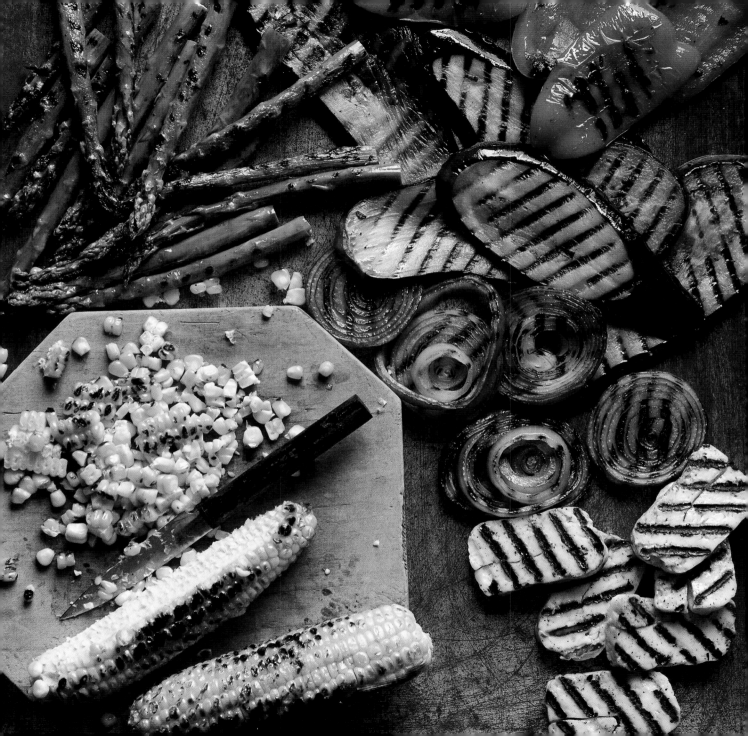

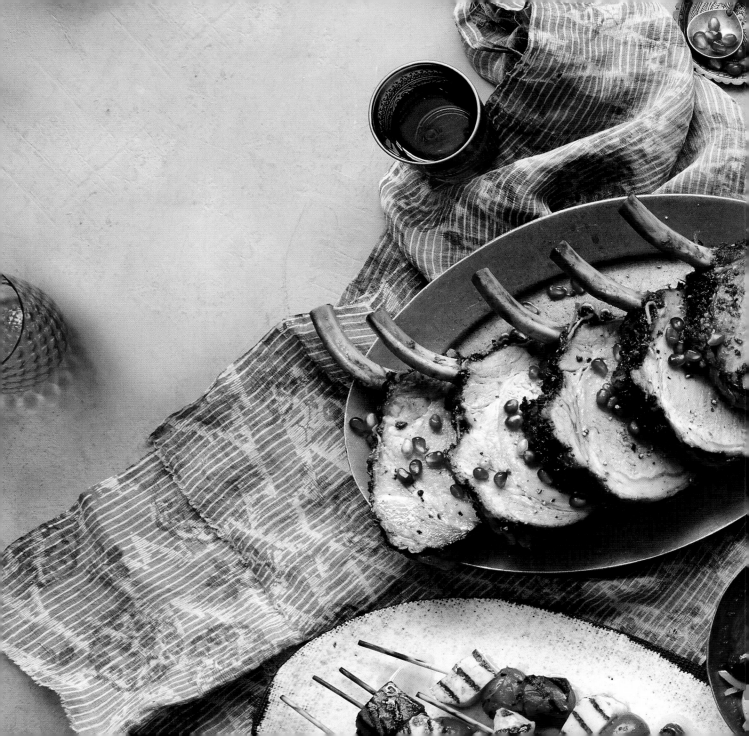

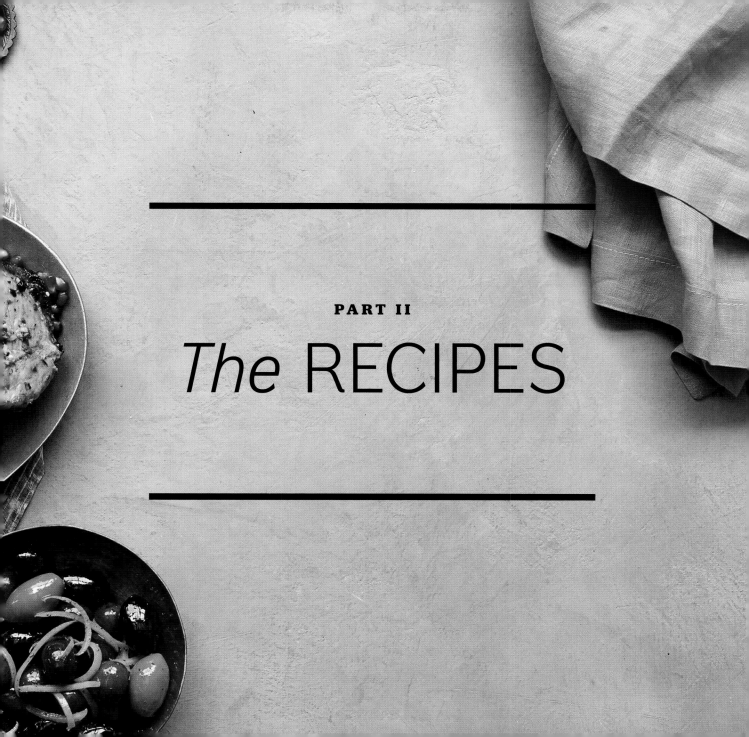

PART II

The RECIPES

Chapter 4
Breakfast

Grabbing a granola bar while you run out the door isn't exactly a pleasant way to start your day, is it? Breakfasts in the Mediterranean tend to be light—often, just coffee with milk, bread with fruit and cheese, or a poached egg—and they aren't rushed. As with larger lunches and dinners, Mediterranean eaters make it a point to have their morning bite sitting down, in the company of others.

Why? Because taking even just a few minutes to pull together a simple meal and enjoy it while sitting at the table sets the tone for your entire morning—and can spell the difference between calm and chaos in the hours ahead.

That's not all. Eating at the table instead of while you're on the go could minimize dis-tractions and help you to eat less overall, British findings suggest.[1] And with recipes *this* delicious, you'll want to make sure you're fully present so you can enjoy every bite. Even if breakfast can't be a sit-down event every single day, these tips can help you make it happen more often.

• **PLAN YOUR BREAKFAST MENUS.** What's for breakfast this upcoming week? If your usual answer is *I don't know yet*, it might be time to make a change. On the weekend, sit down and decide on your morning meals for the upcoming week. Think about what would be the most satisfying to you, but also take the time to consider what works best for your schedule. Opt for fast, no-cook meals (or ones that can be prepped ahead of time) on days when you know you have to be out the door

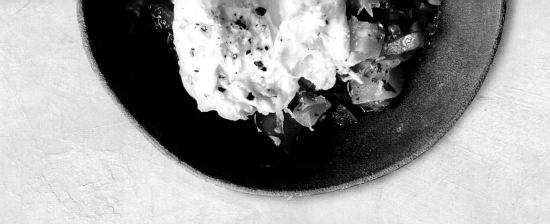

earlier, like Labneh-Avocado Toast with Anchovy Crumbles (page 85) or Savory Cottage Cheese Breakfast Bowl (page 69). Save the slower, more involved items for those mornings when you know you'll have a bit more time.

• **PREP YOUR MEALS IN ADVANCE.** Once you have your breakfasts planned out, figure out which of your meals (if any) require advance prep. Things like frittatas, whole grain muffins, or fruit compotes can be made ahead and enjoyed all week long.

• **SET THE TABLE AFTER DINNER.** Put out the plates, bowls, cups, and utensils for tomorrow's breakfast *tonight*. It only takes a few minutes, and it means you'll have one less step standing between you and a stress-free meal in the morning.

• **STREAMLINE YOUR A.M. ROUTINE.** Think about whether there's anything you can cut out that would give you a bit more time for breakfast. For instance, could you get right out of bed instead of spending 10 minutes scrolling through social media? Or lay out your clothes and pack your bag the night before, so you're not scrambling to get your things together before you run out the door?

• **WAKE UP A LITTLE BIT EARLIER.** Sure, it might seem tough at first. But once you see how much calmer your mornings feel, it just might be worth it. Go ahead—give it a try!

Recipes

SAVORY COTTAGE CHEESE BREAKFAST BOWL

This eastern-Mediterranean dish might seem unusual, but think of it as a Greek salad coming to breakfast. Even though it's a low-cal start, the protein-rich cottage cheese will help fill you up, keeping you satiated until lunch rolls around.

PREP TIME: 10 MINUTES / TOTAL TIME: 10 MINUTES / SERVES 4

2   cups low-fat cottage cheese
2   tablespoons chopped mixed fresh herbs,
     such as basil, dill, flat-leaf parsley, and oregano
½   teaspoon ground black pepper
1   large tomato, chopped
1   small cucumber, peeled and chopped
¼   cup pitted kalamata olives, halved
1   tablespoon extra-virgin olive oil

In a medium bowl, combine the cottage cheese, herbs, and pepper. Add the tomato, cucumber, and olives and gently stir to combine. Drizzle with the oil to serve.

Per serving: 181 calories, 15 g protein, 8 g carbohydrates, 5 g sugars, 10 g total fat, 2 g saturated fat, 1 g fiber, 788 mg sodium

ITALIAN VEGETABLE FRITTATA

Frittatas are a wonderful, hearty way to get vegetables in any time of the day. They are also very forgiving: If you don't have one ingredient, just replace it with something else! You can mix and match any vegetables or herbs, and it will still be delicious.

PREP TIME: 10 MINUTES / TOTAL TIME: 35 MINUTES / SERVES 4

2	tablespoons olive oil
1	small onion, chopped
1	small red bell pepper, seeded and chopped
½	zucchini, halved lengthwise and sliced into half-moons
1	cup cherry tomatoes, halved
1	clove garlic, minced
½	teaspoon kosher salt
½	teaspoon ground black pepper
8	eggs
½	teaspoon chopped fresh rosemary

1. Preheat the oven to 375°F.

2. In a medium ovenproof skillet over medium heat, warm the oil until shimmering. Cook the onion, bell pepper, zucchini, tomatoes, garlic, salt, and black pepper, stirring, until the vegetables are tender and the liquid they released has evaporated, about 8 minutes. Meanwhile, whisk the eggs with the rosemary.

3. Pour the eggs over the vegetables and quickly stir to incorporate. Transfer to the oven and bake until the edges brown and the center is just done, about 15 minutes. (A knife inserted in the middle would come out clean.)

Per serving: 232 calories, 14 g protein, 7 g carbohydrates, 4 g sugars, 17 g total fat, 4 g saturated fat, 2 g fiber, 388 mg sodium

NOTE: Mix things up with different combinations.

✻ Artichoke hearts and asparagus
✻ Fennel and potato
✻ Broccoli and leek
✻ Brussels sprouts and pearl onions

70

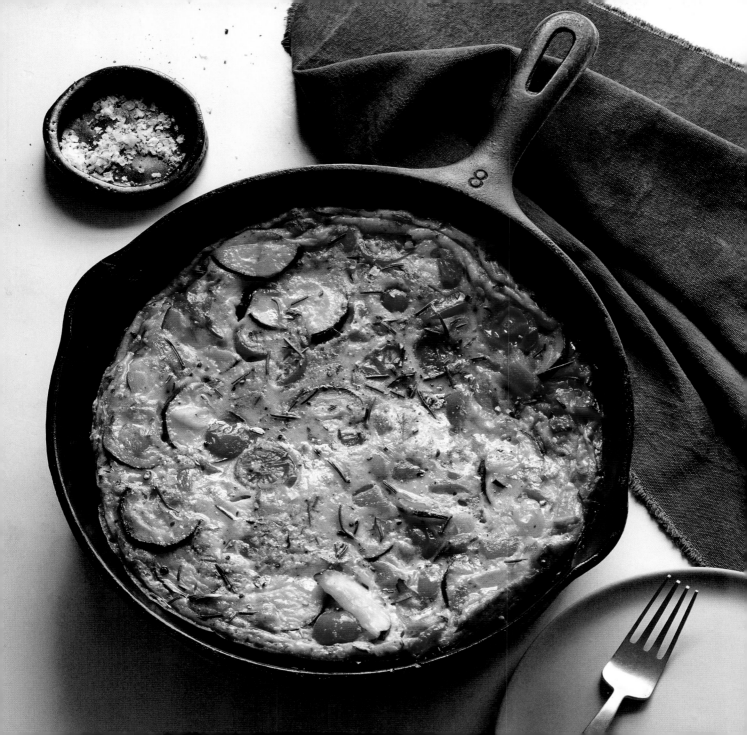

TORTILLA ESPAÑOLA
(SPANISH OMELET)

Traditionally, the potatoes in this Spanish omelet are fried, but baking simplifies the recipe and uses less oil. can be served as breakfast, lunch, dinner, or a snack. It's even great cold the next day—*if* you have leftovers!

PREP TIME: I0 MINUTES / TOTAL TIME: 50 MINUTES / SERVES 4

1½ pounds Yukon gold potatoes, scrubbed and thinly sliced
3 tablespoons olive oil, divided
I teaspoon kosher salt, divided
I sweet white onion, thinly sliced
3 cloves garlic, minced
8 eggs
½ teaspoon ground black pepper

1. Preheat the oven to 350°F. Line 2 baking sheets with parchment paper.

2. In a large bowl, toss the potatoes with 1 tablespoon of the oil and ½ teaspoon of the salt until well coated. Spread over the 2 baking sheets in a single layer. Roast the potatoes, rotating the baking sheets halfway through cooking, until tender but not browned, about 15 minutes. Using a spatula, remove the potatoes from the baking sheets and let cool until warm.

3. Meanwhile, in a medium skillet over medium-low heat, cook the onion in 1 tablespoon of the oil, stirring, until soft and golden, about 10 minutes. Add the garlic and cook until fragrant, about 2 minutes. Transfer the onion and garlic to a plate and let cool until warm.

72

4. In a large bowl, beat the eggs, pepper, and the remaining ½ teaspoon salt vigorously until the yolks and whites are completely combined and slightly frothy. Stir in the potatoes and onion and garlic and combine well, being careful not to break too many potatoes.

5. In the same skillet over medium-high heat, warm the remaining 1 tablespoon oil until shimmering, swirling to cover the whole surface. Pour in the egg mixture and spread the contents evenly. Cook for 1 minute and reduce the heat to medium-low. Cook until the edges of the egg are set and the center is slightly wet, about 8 minutes. Using a spatula, nudge the omelet to make sure it moves freely in the skillet.

6. Place a rimless plate, the size of the skillet, over the omelet. Place one hand over the plate and, in a swift motion, flip the omelet onto the plate. Slide the omelet back into the skillet, cooked side up. Cook until completely set, a toothpick inserted into the middle comes out clean, about 6 minutes.

7. Transfer to a serving plate and let cool for 5 minutes. Serve warm or room temperature.

Per serving: 376 calories, 16 g protein, 36 g carbohydrates, 4 g sugars, 20 g total fat, 5 g saturated fat, 4 g fiber, 678 mg sodium

HOMEMADE RICOTTA CHEESE AND BREAKFAST BOWL

This recipe makes more cheese than you'll need for a breakfast bowl, so use the leftovers any way you'd normally use ricotta: Add herbs and spread it on toast, mix in Parmigiano-Reggiano cheese and stuff it into manicotti shells, stir in powdered sugar and pipe it into cannoli shells, or dollop it plain on a pizza crust. Be sure to use whole milk here—lower-fat milks won't have enough fat to separate into curds and whey. And don't forget to save the whey for use in smoothies.

PREP TIME: 5 MINUTES / TOTAL TIME: I HOUR / MAKES ABOUT 2 CUPS RICOTTA (8 SERVINGS)

RICOTTA CHEESE

½   gallon whole milk (cow's or goat's)
   Generous pinch of kosher salt
2   tablespoons apple cider vinegar or fresh lemon juice

BREAKFAST BOWL

¼   cup Homemade Ricotta Cheese (above)
I   teaspoon honey
2   tablespoons fresh berries of your choice
I   tablespoon sliced almonds, toasted

1. *To make the ricotta cheese:* Set a colander in a large bowl and line with cheesecloth.

2. In a large pot over medium heat, warm the milk and salt to between 195°F and 200°F (do not boil), stirring occasionally, about 15 minutes. Use a candy/deep-fry thermometer to keep an eye on the temperature.

3. Reduce the heat to low and slowly stir in the vinegar or lemon juice, a bit at a time. Look for curdling, or a distinct separation of the milky white solids from the watery, yellowish whey, about 2 minutes. If it's still a milky mixture once you've added all the vinegar or lemon juice, increase the temperature to 205°F until it separates.

RICOTTA

It's good for more than just lasagna or baked ziti. Rich, creamy ricotta and other soft cheeses pair wonderfully with fresh fruit for both breakfast and dessert. And the nutritional benefits are impressive: Half a cup of part-skim ricotta serves up 14 grams of protein along with 337 milligrams of bone-boosting calcium—that's more than a cup of 1% milk. Try topping ricotta with berries and a drizzle of honey for a quick morning meal or scooping a dollop over warm grilled peaches or poached pears for an elegant dessert.

4. With a slotted spoon, carefully transfer the curds into the colander. Pour the remaining curds and whey through the colander, reserving the whey if you like. Drain for 30 to 60 minutes. The longer it drains, the thicker and drier the ricotta.

5. Transfer the ricotta to an airtight container and store in the refrigerator for up to 4 days. Reserve the whey in an airtight container in the refrigerator for up to 1 week. Use it in smoothies, mashed potatoes, or anywhere else you would use milk or buttermilk.

6. *To make the breakfast bowl:* Spoon the ricotta into a bowl. Drizzle with the honey. Top with the berries and almonds.

Per serving (ricotta only): 151 calories, 8 g protein, 12 g carbohydrates, 12 g sugars, 8 g total fat, 4.5 g saturated fat, 0 g fiber, 178 mg sodium

Per serving (breakfast bowl): 215 calories, 9 g protein, 22 g carbohydrates, 19 g sugars, 11 g total fat, 4.5 g saturated fat, 1 g fiber, 178 mg sodium

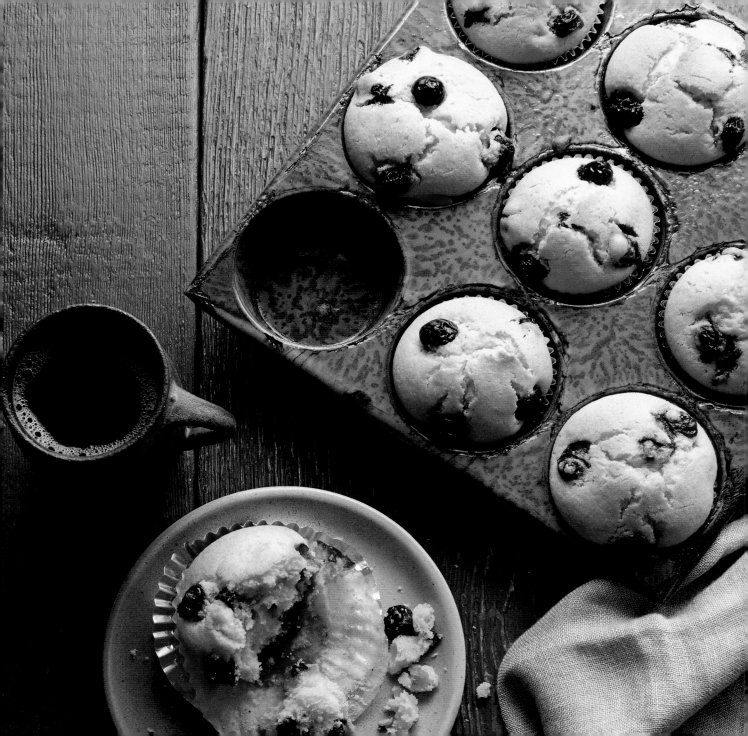

BLUEBERRY-LEMON TEA CAKES

If you've never baked with olive oil before, you're in for a treat: These fruity, lemony cakes are moist and rich without being dense. They're delicious for brunch and decadent enough for dessert.

PREP TIME: 10 MINUTES / TOTAL TIME: 35 MINUTES / SERVES 12

4   eggs
½   cup granulated sugar
    Grated peel of 1 lemon
1½ cups all-purpose flour
¾   cup fine cornmeal
2   teaspoons baking powder
1   teaspoon kosher salt
1   cup extra-virgin olive oil
1½ cups fresh or frozen blueberries

1. Preheat the oven to 350°F. Grease a 12-cup muffin pan or line with paper liners.
2. With an electric mixer set to medium speed, beat the eggs and sugar together until they are pale and fluffy. Stir in the lemon peel.
3. In a medium bowl, stir together the flour, cornmeal, baking powder, and salt. With the mixer on low speed, alternate adding the flour mixture and oil to the egg mixture. Fold in the blueberries.
4. Dollop the batter into the muffin pan. Bake until the tops are golden and a toothpick inserted in the middle comes out clean, 20 to 25 minutes.

Per serving: 332 calories, 5 g protein, 32 g carbohydrates, 10 g sugars, 20 g total fat, 3 g saturated fat, 2 g fiber, 299 mg sodium

77

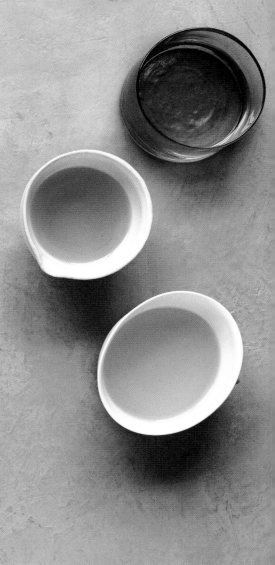

OLIVE OIL

Calling olive oil liquid gold, as the ancient Greeks did,[2] isn't much of an exaggeration. Swapping out saturated fats for monounsaturated ones like olive oil raises levels of HDL, or "good," cholesterol and lowers triglyceride and blood pressure levels, curbing the risk for heart disease and stroke. In fact, a 6-year study that followed nearly 9,000 adults found that those who ate 4 or more tablespoons of extra-virgin olive oil daily had a 30 percent lower risk of having a heart attack or stroke or of dying of heart disease compared to those who followed a low-fat diet.[3]

Why? Olive oil is rich in polyphenols and tocopherols—antioxidant compounds thought to fight harmful inflammation in blood vessels. And pairing olive oil with vegetables like leafy greens, celery, or carrots could make it even more potent. These vegetables contain naturally occurring nitrates and nitrites, which some findings suggest could join forces with olive oil's healthy fats to create beneficial fatty acids that relax blood vessels and lower blood pressure.[4]

This delicious fat does more than just protect your heart, though. Findings show that compounds in olive oil could help sweep away harmful plaque buildup in the brain that contributes to Alzheimer's disease.[5] What's more, eating an olive oil–rich meal appears to raise blood levels of the hormone serotonin, which contributes to feelings of fullness. German study participants who added a drizzle of olive oil to low-fat yogurt daily for 3 months reported feeling more satisfied than those who added an equal amount of lard, butter, or canola oil to their yogurt.[6] Amazingly, even the smell of olive oil alone was enough to significantly boost feelings of satiety. That's one good fat.

FRUIT AND NUT BREAKFAST COUSCOUS

This versatile dish can be altered to suit your tastes. You can substitute any dried fruit for the cranberries and raisins; try figs, dates, or dried blueberries. Or swap out the almonds with your favorite nut.

PREP TIME: 5 MINUTES / TOTAL TIME: 20 MINUTES / SERVES 4

1½   cups 2% milk
1   cup couscous
¼   cup dried cranberries
¼   cup raisins
1   tablespoon honey
1   teaspoon grated orange peel
¼   cup sliced almonds

1. In a medium saucepan, bring the milk to a boil. Remove the saucepan from the heat and stir in the couscous, cranberries, raisins, honey, and orange peel. Cover and let rest for 15 minutes.

2. Fluff the couscous with a fork, and divide among 4 bowls. Top with the almonds and serve.

Per serving: 308 calories, 10 g protein, 57 g carbohydrates, 19 g sugars, 5 g total fat, 1 g saturated fat, 4 g fiber, 49 mg sodium

79

CHICKPEA-POTATO HASH WITH FRIED EGGS

This brunch favorite gets a flavorful Mediterranean spin with summer vegetables, chickpeas, and plenty of herbs.

PREP TIME: 10 MINUTES / TOTAL TIME: 30 MINUTES / SERVES 4

3   tablespoons olive oil, divided
2   russet potatoes, scrubbed and diced
1   onion, diced
1   zucchini, diced
1   clove garlic, minced
½   teaspoon dried oregano
½   teaspoon kosher salt
½   teaspoon ground black pepper, plus more for serving
1   pint cherry tomatoes
1   can (15 ounces) chickpeas, drained and rinsed (see note)
½   cup chopped fresh flat-leaf parsley
8   eggs

1. In a large skillet over medium heat, warm 1 tablespoon of the oil. Cook the potatoes and onion, stirring constantly, until the onion is translucent and the potatoes are starting to get tender, about 7 minutes. Stir in the zucchini, garlic, oregano, salt, and pepper and cook until the zucchini begins to brown, about 5 minutes. Add the tomatoes, chickpeas, and parsley and stir to combine. Reduce the heat to low and cook until heated through, about 5 minutes.

2. Meanwhile, in another large skillet over medium heat, warm the remaining 2 tablespoons oil. Crack the eggs into the skillet, keeping them separate. Cover and cook until the whites are set but the yolks are still soft, about 4 minutes. Sprinkle with pepper and serve over the hash.

Per serving: 398 calories, 20 g protein, 33 g carbohydrates, 5 g sugars, 22 g total fat, 5 g saturated fat, 7 g fiber, 606 mg sodium

NOTE: Don't discard that drained liquid. Known as aquafaba (bean water), this stuff is liquid gold! You can use it as a vegan egg substitute to make desserts, condiments, and even cocktails.

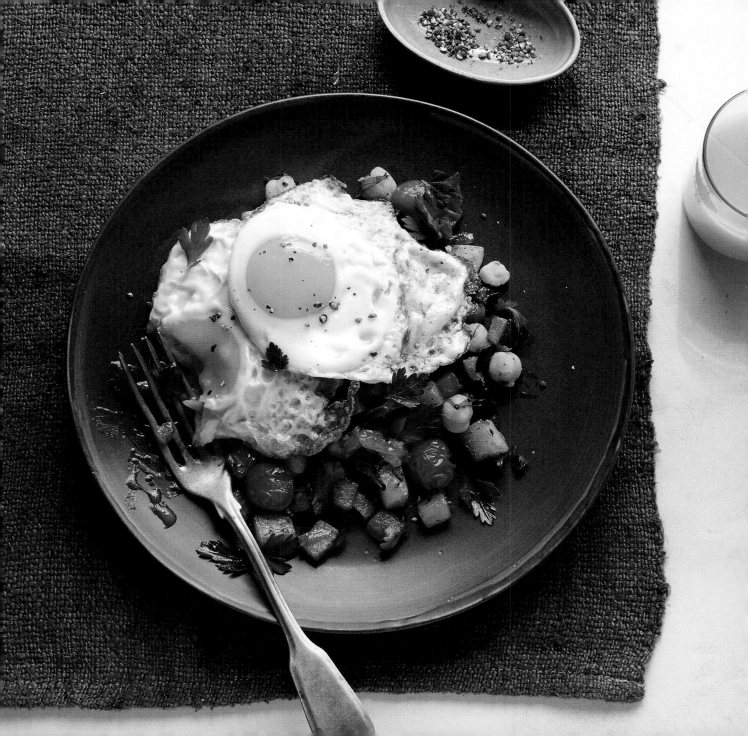

BLACK OLIVE TOAST WITH HERBED HUMMUS

This dressed-up toast comes together in minutes—which means you get a bit more time to sit down and enjoy your meal. For even faster morning prep, make the herbed hummus the night before.

PREP TIME: 5 MINUTES / TOTAL TIME: 10 MINUTES / SERVES 2

¼ cup Hummus (page 149) or store-bought plain hummus

2 tablespoons finely chopped fresh flat-leaf parsley

1 tablespoon finely chopped fresh dill

1 tablespoon finely chopped fresh mint

1 teaspoon finely grated lemon peel

2 slices (½" thick) black olive bread

1 clove garlic, halved

1 tablespoon extra-virgin olive oil

1. In a small bowl, combine the hummus, herbs, and lemon peel.

2. Toast the bread. Immediately rub the warm bread with the garlic.

3. Spread half the hummus over each slice of bread and drizzle with the oil.

Per serving: 276 calories, 8 g protein, 35 g carbohydrates, 5 g sugars, 13 g total fat, 2 g saturated fat, 3 g fiber, 419 mg sodium

82

GARLICKY BEANS AND GREENS WITH POLENTA

Beans, greens, and polenta come together to make a satisfying savory breakfast. For an even heartier meal, put an egg on it!

PREP TIME: 5 MINUTES / TOTAL TIME: 25 MINUTES / SERVES 4

2   tablespoons olive oil, divided
I   roll (18 ounces) precooked polenta, cut into ½"-thick slices
4   cloves garlic, minced
4   cups chopped greens, such as kale, mustard greens, collards, or chard
2   tomatoes, seeded and diced
I   can (15 ounces) small white beans, drained and rinsed (see note on page 80)
     Kosher salt and ground black pepper, to taste

1. In a large skillet over medium heat, warm 1 tablespoon of the oil. Cook the polenta slices, flipping once, until golden and crispy, about 5 minutes per side. Remove the polenta and keep warm.

2. Add the remaining 1 tablespoon oil to the skillet. Cook the garlic until softened, 1 minute. Add the greens, tomatoes, and beans and cook until the greens are wilted and bright green and the beans are heated through, 10 minutes. Season to taste with the salt and pepper. To serve, top the polenta with the beans and greens.

Per serving: 231 calories, 11 g protein, 39 g carbohydrates, 2 g sugar, 4 g fat, 1 g saturated fat, 6 g fiber, 235 mg sodium

83

LEAFY GREENS

When it comes to Mediterranean-style foods with brain-protecting benefits, leafy greens are some of the best of the bunch. They are the top sources of lutein—a phytonutrient that protects structures in the brain and supports healthy cognitive function[7]—and other brain healthy nutrients, including vitamin K, beta-carotene, and folate. Kale, spinach, arugula, chard, and collards are all great options, so pick the ones you love and give them a regular spot on the table. Findings suggest that I to 2 servings per day may be optimal.[8] And if you're lucky enough to come across wild greens like dandelion greens, nettles, or purslane—scoop them up! They're a tasty, nutrient-rich alternative to the usual picks, and it's common for Greeks to enjoy them simply boiled and drizzled with olive oil and lemon juice.

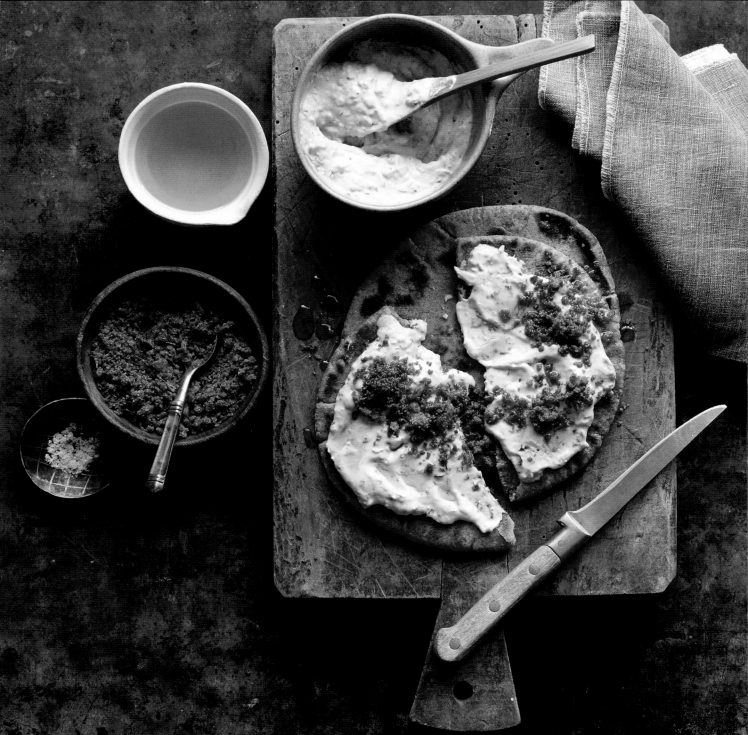

LABNEH-AVOCADO TOAST WITH ANCHOVY CRUMBLES

Anchovies for breakfast? Cooking up the anchovies helps mellow out their fishiness and adds a great protein boost.

PREP TIME: 5 MINUTES / TOTAL TIME: 10 MINUTES / SERVES 2

½   jar (3.5–4.5 ounces) anchovies in oil
1   tablespoon whole wheat flour
½   ripe avocado
¼   cup labneh or low-fat plain Greek yogurt
2   tablespoons fresh lemon juice
1   tablespoon thinly sliced fresh chives
1   teaspoon finely chopped fresh tarragon
½   teaspoon fresh thyme leaves
    Pinch of kosher salt
    Pinch of ground black pepper
2   Whole Wheat Pitas (page 164)
1   tablespoon extra-virgin olive oil

1. In a small skillet, add half the anchovies from the jar with half their oil and the flour. Cook over medium heat, breaking the anchovies up with a wooden spoon until small crumbles form, about 5 minutes. Continue to cook until crisp, about 2 minutes.

2. Meanwhile, in a medium bowl, mash the avocado with the labneh or yogurt, lemon juice, herbs, salt, and pepper.

3. Warm the pitas in a skillet, toaster, or oven. Top with the avocado mash, sprinkle with the anchovies, and drizzle with the olive oil.

Per serving: 380 calories, 14 g protein, 45 g carbohydrates, 2 g sugars, 17 g total fat, 2 g saturated fat, 7 g fiber, 1,483 mg sodium

85

LABNEH

Like Greek yogurt? Then chances are you'll love labneh, a fermented dairy food that's a staple in Lebanese and Israeli cooking. Made by straining full-fat yogurt for several hours, labneh is a thick, cream cheese–like spread that's richer and tangier than yogurt. It's delicious as a meze topped with chopped vegetables and drizzled with olive oil. Plus just like yogurt, it's packed with protein and beneficial probiotics.

MEDITERRANEAN MUESLI AND BREAKFAST BOWL

Unlike granola, which is baked, muesli is an uncooked combination of oats, fruits, nuts, and seeds—without the added sugar and oil used to bind granola together. With origins in the mountains of Switzerland, this muesli has a Mediterranean spin on it with the addition of dried figs, dates, and pistachios. We've also added wheat or rye flakes and oat bran to boost the whole-grain nutrition—look for them in the natural foods section of the supermarket.

PREP TIME: 10 MINUTES / TOTAL TIME: 10 MINUTES / MAKES ABOUT 6 CUPS MUESLI (12 SERVINGS)

MUESLI

- 3 cups old-fashioned rolled oats
- 1 cup wheat or rye flakes
- 1 cup pistachios or almonds, coarsely chopped
- ½ cup oat bran
- 8 dried apricots, chopped
- 8 dates, chopped
- 8 dried figs, chopped

BREAKFAST BOWL

- ½ cup Mediterranean Muesli (above)
- 1 cup low-fat plain Greek yogurt or milk
- 2 tablespoons pomegranate seeds (optional)
- ½ teaspoon black or white sesame seeds

1. *To make the muesli:* In a medium bowl, combine the oats, wheat or rye flakes, pistachios or almonds, oat bran, apricots, dates, and figs. Transfer to an airtight container and store for up to 1 month.

2. *To make the breakfast bowl:* In a bowl, combine the muesli with the yogurt or milk. Top with the pomegranate seeds, if using, and the sesame seeds.

Per serving (muesli only): 234 calories, 8 g protein, 40 g carbohydrates, 16 g sugars, 6 g total fat, 0.5 g saturated fat, 6 g fiber, 54 mg sodium

Per serving (breakfast bowl): 393 calories, 27 g protein, 50 g carbohydrates, 25 g sugars, 12 g total fat, 4 g saturated fat, 6 g fiber, 130 mg sodium

NOTE: Muesli and milk may be gently heated over medium heat for a warming breakfast. Or mix yogurt into a serving of muesli and leave in the refrigerator overnight for a creamier, raw version in the morning.

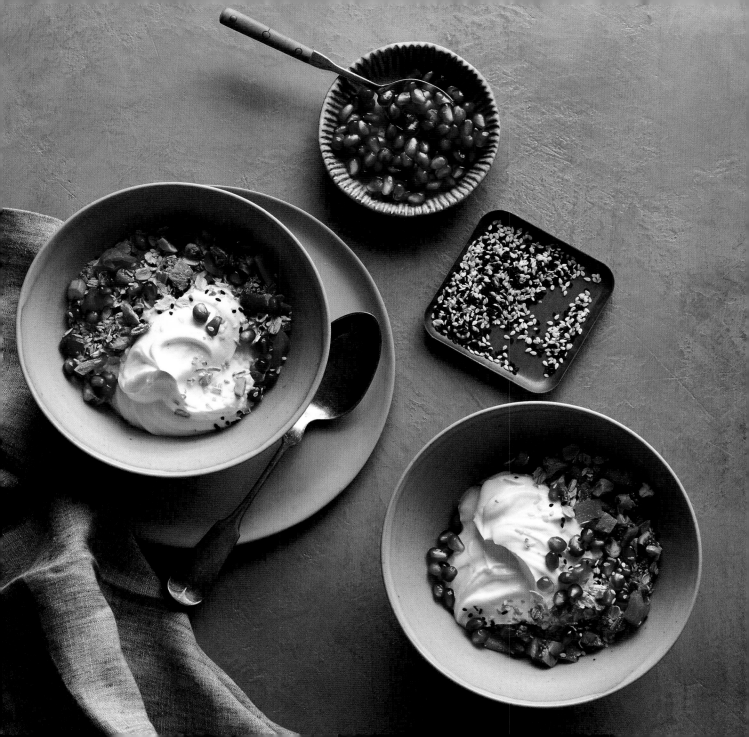

Chapter 5
Soups, Salads, and Sandwiches

Lunch is the main meal of the day in many Mediterranean countries, and it tends to be pretty leisurely. In places like Italy or Spain, it's not uncommon for lunch to last for 2 hours or more and consist of multiple courses. Sounds like pure luxury! Here at home, hours-long midday meals simply aren't realistic for most people.

But that's okay! If you're used to plowing through a deli sandwich while dashing off e-mails or reading reports, even carving out 15 or 20 minutes for lunch will feel like a real treat. Especially when you bring along one of the fresh, tasty dishes in this chapter.

What's the big deal about making time for lunch, anyway? For starters, dining away from your desk minimizes interruptions that can make you stressed out or distracted, like the nonstop ding of your inbox. The same goes for stay-at-home parents who eat one-handed, standing over the sink and even as they lovingly pack their child's meal. You need a chance to reset and refill your tank so you have more energy to tackle everything on your afternoon to-do list. And though it might seem impossible now, finding a few spare moments for a quiet, work-free or chore-free lunch is easier than you think. Here's how to make it happen.

- **BLOCK OUT YOUR LUNCHES.** Pick a time period for lunch and put it on your calendar. Having a break already built into the schedule means you'll be less likely to skip it, and it reminds others not to disturb you. If you're worried that putting lunch on your calendar might look bad to coworkers, consider blocking off the time as research or brainstorming sessions.

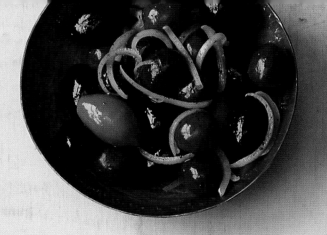

- **FIND A DEDICATED DINING SPOT.** It could be a bench in the park when the weather's nice or the communal break room when it's cold or dark. Eating somewhere—anywhere!—that isn't your desk is one of the simplest ways to jolt yourself out of work mode. And over time, your brain will start to associate this go-to spot as a place where you relax and recharge. If you are at home, clear the laundry off that table or special bench you put in your backyard but never sit on.

- **BRING YOUR LUNCH FROM HOME.** Homemade lunches are, of course, cheaper and healthier than restaurant meals. But they also add precious time to your lunch break because you don't have to spend 10 minutes (or more) running down to the corner deli and waiting for your order. You are also more likely to select healthier choices the night before than if you are hungry and faced with a restaurant or cafeteria menu.

- **STOW AWAY YOUR DEVICES.** You *know* you'll still be tempted to check your phone even if it's switched to silent mode. So avoid taking it, along with your tablet or laptop, with you to lunch whenever possible. Most messages aren't so urgent that they require an immediate response. If you're still worried about being MIA, put up an away message letting people know that you've received their note and will reply when you're back at your desk.

- **SCHEDULE LUNCHTIME MEETINGS.** On hectic days when there just isn't time for a break, try to make meetings happen over lunch. Chances are spending your meal chatting with a coworker or client will be more enjoyable than eating solo by the glow of your screen.

Recipes

SOUPS

SALADS

SANDWICHES

AVGOLEMONO
(EGG LEMON) SOUP

Avgo (egg) *lemono* (lemon) soup is a classic in Greece. It's velvety and smooth, and with the addition of chicken, rice, and peas, it makes for a lovely, filling soup. Using leftover brown rice and rotisserie chicken make this a quick weeknight meal.

PREP TIME: 10 MINUTES / TOTAL TIME: 25 MINUTES / SERVES 4

1 tablespoon olive oil
1 shallot, finely chopped
6 cups low-sodium chicken broth
¼ cup fresh lemon juice
3 eggs
3 cups baby spinach
1 cup cooked brown rice
1 cup shredded cooked chicken
Kosher salt and ground black pepper, to taste
2 tablespoons chopped fresh dill

1. In a large saucepan over medium heat, warm the oil until shimmering. Cook the shallot, stirring, until softened, about 5 minutes. Add the broth and lemon juice and bring to a simmer.

2. In a medium bowl, whisk the eggs. Using a ladle, pour a spoonful of the broth into the eggs while whisking. Reduce the heat to low and whisk the egg mixture into the broth in the saucepan.

3. Add the spinach, rice, and chicken and cook until warmed through and the spinach is wilted, about 5 minutes. Season to taste with the salt and pepper. Serve with the dill sprinkled on top.

Per serving: 355 calories, 33 g protein, 31 g carbohydrates, 2 g sugars, 11 g total fat, 3 g saturated fat, 3 g fiber, 304 mg sodium

CRANBERRY BEAN MINESTRONE

Cranberry beans, also called borlotti or Roman beans, are a cream-colored bean with lovely red swirls. If you prefer to use dry beans, add them to the slow cooker with the vegetables. If you don't have a slow cooker, see the stove-top cooking method in the note below.

PREP TIME: I5 MINUTES / TOTAL TIME: 3 HOURS 45 MINUTES / SERVES 6

I   quart low-sodium vegetable broth
I   can (I4.5 ounces) diced tomatoes
2   carrots, thinly sliced
2   ribs celery, thinly sliced
I   onion, chopped
3   cloves garlic, sliced
I   tablespoon dried oregano
I   bay leaf
½   teaspoon kosher salt
½   teaspoon ground black pepper
2   cans (I5 ounces each) cranberry beans, drained and rinsed (see note on page 80)
I   small zucchini, halved lengthwise and sliced ¼" thick
I½ cups whole grain ditalini or elbow pasta
6   tablespoons finely grated Parmigiano-Reggiano cheese
3   tablespoons shredded fresh basil

1. In a 4- or 6-quart slow cooker, combine the broth, tomatoes, carrots, celery, onion, garlic, oregano, bay leaf, salt, and pepper. Cover and cook until the vegetables are tender, on low 6 to 8 hours or high 3 to 4 hours.

2. Remove the cover and add the beans, zucchini, and pasta. Cook on high until the pasta is tender, about 30 minutes. Remove the bay leaf and garnish each serving with the cheese and basil.

Per serving: 256 calories, 14 g protein, 43 g carbohydrates, 6 g sugars, 3 g total fat, 1 g saturated fat, 11 g fiber, 924 mg sodium

NOTE: To cook the minestrone on the stove, in a large soup pot, heat 2 tablespoons olive oil. Cook the carrots, celery, and onion over medium-high until softened, 5 minutes. Add the garlic, oregano, bay leaf, salt, and pepper and cook for 1 minute. Add the broth and tomatoes and bring to a boil. Cover, reduce the heat to a simmer, and cook until the vegetables are tender, about 30 minutes. Add the beans, zucchini, and pasta and cook until the pasta is al dente, about 10 minutes.

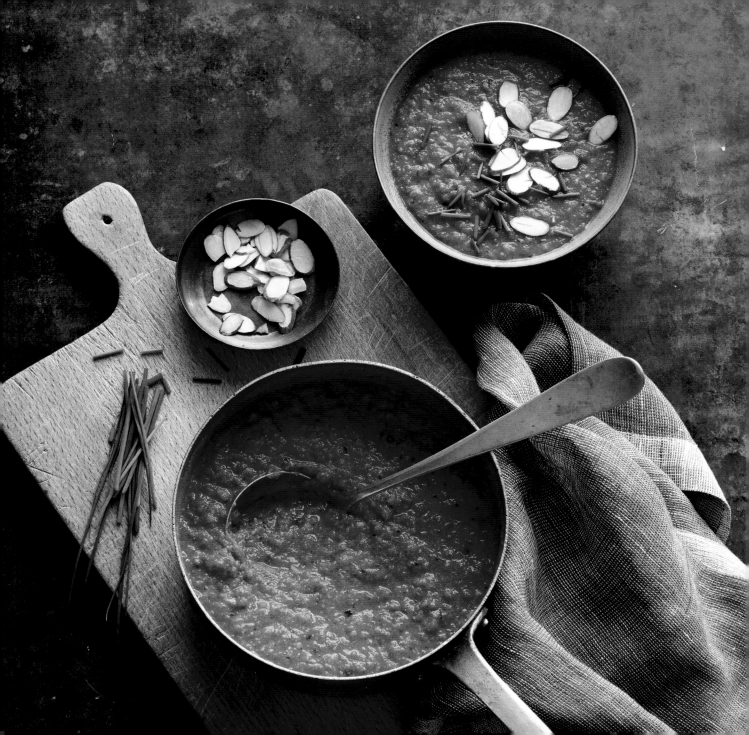

ROMESCO SOUP

Named for the famed Spanish sauce, we use the same flavors and nuts as a thickener for the soup.

PREP TIME: 5 MINUTES / TOTAL TIME: 25 MINUTES / SERVES 6

1 tablespoon olive oil
1 onion, chopped
1 teaspoon kosher salt
6 cloves garlic, minced
½ teaspoon paprika
2 jars (12 ounces each) roasted red peppers, drained and chopped
1 can (28 ounces) diced fire-roasted tomatoes
1 cup low-sodium chicken broth
½ cup almond meal (see note)
1 tablespoon balsamic vinegar
¼ teaspoon ground black pepper
¼ cup sliced almonds, toasted
  Chopped chives, for garnish

1. In a large pot over medium-high heat, warm the oil. Cook the onion and salt, stirring occasionally, until the onion is soft, 5 minutes.

2. Add the garlic and cook until soft, 2 minutes. Stir in the paprika and cook until fragrant, 1 minute. Add the peppers, tomatoes, and broth. Bring to a boil, reduce the heat to a simmer, cover, and cook until heated through, 15 minutes.

3. Add the almond meal and vinegar. With an immersion blender or a regular blender in batches, puree the soup until smooth. Stir in the pepper and serve topped with a sprinkle of the almonds and chives.

Per serving: 162 calories, 5 g protein, 17 g carbohydrates, 9 g sugars, 9 g total fat, 1 g saturated fat, 4 g fiber, 701 mg sodium

NOTE: If you can't find almond meal, pulse 4 ounces raw almonds in a food processor until very fine. Be careful not to overprocess or you will have almond butter instead.

RED, WHITE, AND GREEN GAZPACHOS

This Spanish cold soup can be made in many ways, depending on where you are from in Spain. Here are three of our favorites.

PREP TIME: 15 MINUTES / TOTAL TIME: 4 HOURS 20 MINUTES / SERVES 6

RED GAZPACHO

- 1½ pounds ripe red tomatoes, cut into large pieces
- 1 large green bell pepper, seeded and coarsely chopped
- 2 slices whole wheat bread, left out overnight to dry
- 3 cloves garlic, coarsely chopped
- ⅓ cup extra-virgin olive oil
- 2 tablespoons sherry vinegar
- 1 teaspoons kosher salt
- 1 teaspoon ground black pepper

Per serving: 157 calories, 3 g protein, 10 g carbohydrates, 4 g sugars, 13 g total fat, 2 g saturated fat, 3 g fiber, 364 mg sodium

WHITE GAZPACHO

- 2 large English cucumbers, peeled, seeded, and coarsely chopped
- 2 slices white bread, crusts removed and soaked in ½ cup water for 5 minutes
- 1 shallot, coarsely chopped
- ¼ cup slivered almonds, toasted
- ¼ cup extra-virgin olive oil
- 2 tablespoons champagne vinegar or white wine vinegar
- 2 tablespoons fresh lemon juice
- 2 cloves garlic, coarsely chopped
- ½ teaspoon kosher salt

Per serving: 150 calories, 3 g protein, 9 g carbohydrates, 2 g sugars, 12 g total fat, 2 g saturated fat, 1 g fiber, 196 mg sodium

96

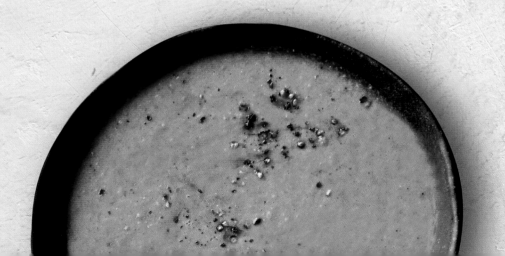

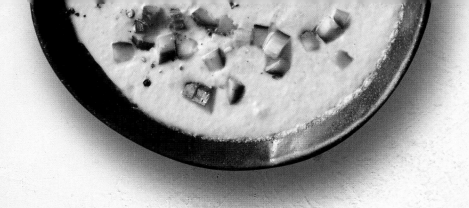

GREEN GAZPACHO

2 large English cucumbers, seeded and coarsely chopped

1 large yellow bell pepper, seeded and coarsely chopped

1 ripe avocado

6 scallions, coarsely chopped

2 slices white bread, crusts removed and coarsely chopped

½ cup chopped mixed fresh herbs, such as flat-leaf parsley, cilantro, mint, and basil

¼ cup extra-virgin olive oil

2 tablespoons red wine vinegar

2 cloves garlic, coarsely chopped

1 teaspoon kosher salt

Per serving: 188 calories, 4 g protein, 13 g carbohydrates, 3 g sugars, 15 g total fat, 2 g saturated fat, 5 g fiber, 375 mg sodium

FOR SERVING (OPTIONAL)

Extra-virgin olive oil, for drizzling

Diced cucumber

Thinly sliced scallions

Freshly ground black pepper

Chopped fresh herbs

In a food processor or blender, combine all the ingredients and puree until smooth. Pass through a medium-mesh sieve and refrigerate until cold, about 4 hours. Season to taste with salt, pepper, and vinegar before serving with the optional toppings.

97

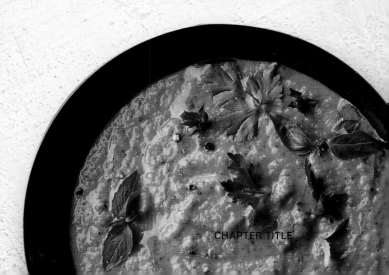

HARIRA
(MOROCCAN CHICKPEA AND LENTIL SOUP)

Harira is to Morocco what chicken noodle soup is to the United States. Eaten throughout the year, but most frequently during the month of Ramadan, harira's beauty lies in its complex flavors derived from simple ingredients. To eat this soup in the traditional manner, enjoy it with friends and family, with bowls of dates, dried figs, fresh herbs, and a honey-kissed dessert such as Tahini Baklava Cups on page 257 or Loukoumades (*Honey Dumplings*) on page 253. The recipe easily halves, if serving a smaller group.

PREP TIME: 20 MINUTES / TOTAL TIME: I HOUR 30 MINUTES / SERVES 8 TO I0

3   tablespoons olive oil
I   yellow onion, finely chopped
2   ribs celery (with leaves), finely chopped
2   carrots, finely chopped
5   cloves garlic, minced
I   tablespoon grated fresh ginger
2   teaspoons turmeric
I½ teaspoons ground cinnamon
I   teaspoon kosher salt
I   teaspoon ground black pepper
    Generous pinch of saffron (about 20 threads)

2   quarts low-sodium chicken broth
I   can (28 ounces) diced tomatoes
½   cup brown rice
2   cups brown lentils, rinsed
2   cans (I5 ounces each) chickpeas or fava beans, drained and rinsed (see note on page 80)
I   cup chopped fresh cilantro, plus more for serving
I   cup chopped fresh flat-leaf parsley, plus more for serving
I–2 tablespoons harissa
2   lemons, cut into wedges
    Low-fat plain Greek yogurt, for serving (optional)

HARISSA

If you're a fan of bold flavors, you'll love this spicy paste made from roasted red and hot chili peppers, garlic, and spices like cumin, saffron, and coriander. Harissa is a staple in North African cooking, where it's often used as a meat rub, and in soups, stews, and cousous. But it's delicious on just about anything—from hummus, to roasted vegetables, to salad dressing, to scrambled eggs. Find harissa in jars, tubes, or cans in the ethnic section of most grocery stores, or in specialty stores or Middle Eastern markets.

1. In a large soup pot over medium heat, warm the oil. Cook the onion, celery, and carrots until the vegetables are tender and begin to take on color, 7 to 8 minutes.

2. Reduce the heat to low and add the garlic, ginger, turmeric, cinnamon, salt, pepper, and saffron. Cook, stirring constantly, until fragrant, 1 minute.

3. Add the broth, tomatoes, and rice. Bring to a boil, reduce the heat to a simmer, cover, and cook for 10 minutes. Add the lentils and chickpeas or fava beans and simmer until the lentils and rice are tender, about 35 minutes. The soup is meant to be thick, but if it seems too thick, add water, $\frac{1}{2}$ cup at a time, to reach desired consistency.

4. Stir in the cilantro, parsley, and harissa and cook for 5 minutes.

5. Garnish each serving with more herbs plus the lemon wedges. Dollop with the yogurt, if using.

Per serving: 406 calories, 23 g protein, 61 g carbohydrates, 6 g sugars, 9 g total fat, 1.5 g saturated fat, 21 g fiber, 833 mg sodium

NOTE: This soup easily transforms into a nonvegetarian dish. Brown $\frac{3}{4}$ pound cubed beef, lamb, or chicken in a bit of oil in the soup pot before cooking the vegetables. Remove and return it to the pot with the lentils.

RIBOLLITA
(TUSCAN BEAN, BREAD, AND VEGETABLE STEW)

This soup is traditionally meant to be prepared one day and then reheated the next day. You can do that, but it is delicious right from the stove, too. If you have a Parmigiano-Reggiano rind, cut off a 2" piece and add it to the soup for more flavor.

PREP TIME: 10 MINUTES / TOTAL TIME: 50 MINUTES / SERVES 6

1 tablespoon olive oil
1 onion, chopped
1 carrot, chopped
1 rib celery, chopped
2 cloves garlic, minced
1 tablespoon fresh rosemary leaves
1 tablespoon fresh thyme leaves
½ teaspoon salt
¼ teaspoon ground black pepper
1 quart low-sodium chicken broth or vegetable broth
1 can (14.5 ounces) diced tomatoes
1 can (15 ounces) white beans, drained and rinsed (see note on page 80)
4 cups chopped kale
2 cups stale whole grain bread cubes
Parmigiano-Reggiano cheese, for garnish

1. In a large soup pot over medium heat, warm the oil. Cook the onion, carrot, and celery until softened, 5 minutes. Stir in the garlic, rosemary, thyme, salt, and pepper and cook for 1 minute.

2. Stir in the broth and tomatoes and bring to a boil. Reduce the heat to a simmer and cook for 30 minutes.

3. Add the beans and kale and cook until the kale has wilted and the beans are heated through, 5 minutes. Remove the soup from the heat and stir in the bread cubes. Serve immediately with a sprinkle of the cheese, or cool to room temperature before storing in the refrigerator.

Per serving: 193 calories, 11 g protein, 30 g carbohydrates, 5 g sugars, 4 g total fat, 1 g saturated fat, 6 g fiber, 501 mg sodium

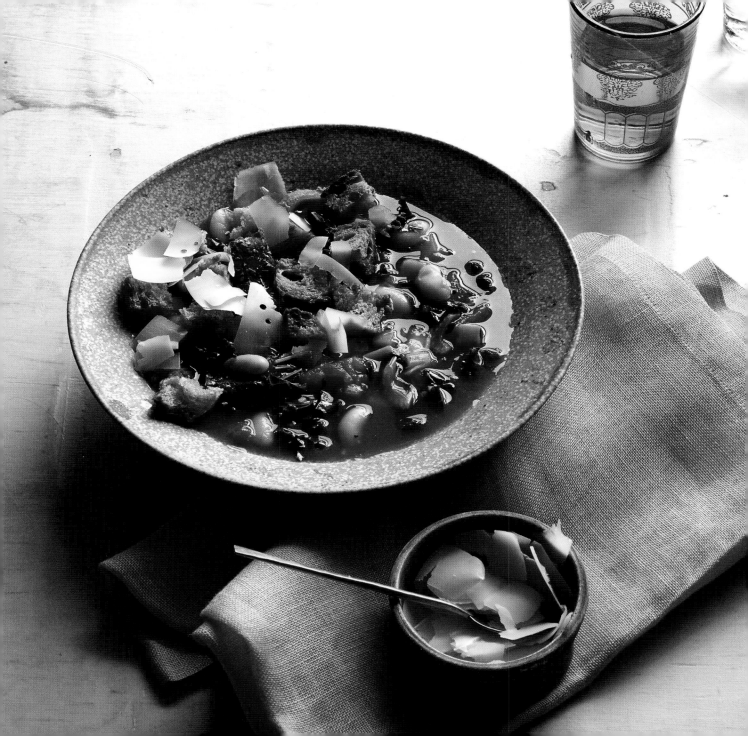

TURKISH RED LENTIL BRIDE SOUP

This soup is traditionally served to new brides right before their weddings to sustain them for what lies ahead.

PREP TIME: 5 MINUTES / TOTAL TIME: I HOUR IO MINUTES / SERVES 4

2 tablespoons olive oil
I yellow onion, finely chopped
½ teaspoon hot paprika, plus more to taste
½ cup red lentils, rinsed
⅓ cup bulgur wheat
I tablespoon tomato paste
I quart low-sodium chicken broth or vegetable broth
¼ cup chopped fresh mint
2 tablespoons fresh lemon juice
Kosher salt, to taste

1. In a large saucepan over medium heat, warm the oil until shimmering. Cook the onion, stirring, until golden, about 10 minutes.
2. Stir in the paprika, lentils, and bulgur to coat in the oil. Add the tomato paste and cook, stirring, until the color darkens, about 2 minutes.
3. Add the broth and bring to a boil. Reduce the heat to a simmer and cook, stirring occasionally to avoid sticking, until the lentils and bulgur are tender and creamy, about 40 minutes.
4. Stir in the mint and lemon juice. Season to taste with the salt.

Per serving: 206 calories, 9 g protein, 27 g carbohydrates, 2 g sugars, 8 g total fat, 1 g saturated fat, 7 g fiber, 139 mg sodium

SICILIAN FISH SOUP

Serve this northern Sicilian *zuppa di pesce* with a crusty bread to sop up every last drop. The recipe easily doubles, and feel free to swap any of the seafood with your favorite varieties, estimating 6 ounces per person.

PREP TIME: 20 MINUTES / TOTAL TIME: 1 HOUR / SERVES 4

3   tablespoons olive oil
1   white onion, chopped
1   bulb fennel, trimmed, cored, and chopped
2   tomatoes, chopped
2   cloves garlic, minced
¼–½ teaspoon red-pepper flakes
2   cups water
⅔   cup dry white wine or water
¾   teaspoon kosher salt
1   pound mussels, scrubbed and debearded (see note)
½   pound shrimp, peeled and deveined
½   pound skin-off white fish, such as cod, halibut, or haddock, cut into 2" chunks
¼   cup chopped fresh flat-leaf parsley
1   lemon, cut into wedges

1. In a medium soup pot over medium heat, warm the oil. Cook the onion and fennel, stirring occasionally, until tender but not browned, 5 to 6 minutes.

2. Add the tomatoes, garlic, and pepper flakes. Cook, stirring occasionally, until the tomatoes begin to break down, 3 to 4 minutes. Add the water, wine or water, and salt and bring to a boil. Reduce the heat to a simmer and cook, stirring occasionally, to blend the flavors and soften the vegetables, about 15 minutes.

3. Add the mussels, shrimp, and fish. Cover and simmer until the shrimp and fish are cooked through and the mussels have opened (discard any that do not), 6 to 8 minutes. Stir in the parsley and serve with the lemon wedges.

Per serving: 299 calories, 25 g protein, 14 g carbohydrates, 3 g sugars, 13 g total fat, 2 g saturated fat, 3 g fiber, 948 mg sodium

NOTE: The beard is the mossy-looking bit that hangs off the mussel where the 2 shells join. It's not inedible, but it is a bit unpleasant. Not every mussel will have a beard, and all it takes is a little tug to pull it free. Tug down, toward the hinge of the mussel, and give it a wiggle to free it.

CROATIAN CABBAGE SOUP

This simple soup is a great example of using meat as a garnish or flavor enhancer. There's only a small amount of bacon here—but its deep, smoky flavor really makes this simple soup shine.

PREP TIME: 10 MINUTES / TOTAL TIME: 45 MINUTES / SERVES 6

6   slices bacon
1   onion, chopped
1   clove garlic, minced
1   red or green bell pepper, seeded and chopped
1   can (28 ounces) diced tomatoes
4   cups shredded green cabbage
4   cups water
1   teaspoon kosher salt
½   teaspoon smoked paprika
½   teaspoon chopped fresh rosemary

1. In a large soup pot over medium heat, cook the bacon until crispy, about 8 minutes. Remove the bacon from the pot and drain on a paper towel–lined plate. Pour out all but 2 tablespoons of the bacon fat from the pot. Crumble the bacon when cool enough to handle.

2. Add the onion and garlic to the pot and cook until softened, 1 to 2 minutes. Add the pepper and tomatoes, stir, and cook for a few more minutes.

3. Stir in the cabbage, water, salt, paprika, and rosemary. Cover and bring to a boil. Reduce the heat to a simmer and cook until the cabbage is tender, 15 minutes. Serve topped with the crumbled bacon.

Per serving: 127 calories, 4 g protein, 12 g carbohydrates, 7 g sugars, 7 g total fat, 2.5 g saturated fat, 3 g fiber, 553 mg sodium

GREEK SALAD WITH LEMON-OREGANO VINAIGRETTE

Greek salads get a bad rap from diner incarnations of iceberg lettuce drenched in dressing with a stray cherry tomato. Here we lose the greens altogether and focus on the vegetables. If you want to stretch the salad or you enjoy a green, chop a head of romaine and toss it in.

PREP TIME: 15 MINUTES / TOTAL TIME: 30 MINUTES / SERVES 8

½ red onion, thinly sliced
¼ cup extra-virgin olive oil
3 tablespoons fresh lemon juice or red wine vinegar
1 clove garlic, minced
1 teaspoon chopped fresh oregano or ½ teaspoon dried
½ teaspoon ground black pepper
¼ teaspoon kosher salt
4 tomatoes, cut into large chunks
1 large English cucumber, peeled, seeded (if desired), and diced
1 large yellow or red bell pepper, chopped
½ cup pitted kalamata or Niçoise olives, halved
¼ cup chopped fresh flat-leaf parsley
4 ounces Halloumi or feta cheese, cut into ½" cubes

1. In a medium bowl, soak the onion in enough water to cover for 10 minutes.

2. In a small bowl, combine the oil, lemon juice or vinegar, garlic, oregano, black pepper, and salt.

3. Drain the onion and add to a large bowl with the tomatoes, cucumber, bell pepper, olives, and parsley. Gently toss to mix the vegetables.

4. Pour the vinaigrette over the salad. Add the cheese and toss again to distribute.

5. Serve immediately, or chill for up to 30 minutes.

Per serving (pita not included): 190 calories, 5 g protein, 8 g carbohydrates, 3 g sugars, 16 g total fat, 4 g saturated fat, 2 g fiber, 554 mg sodium

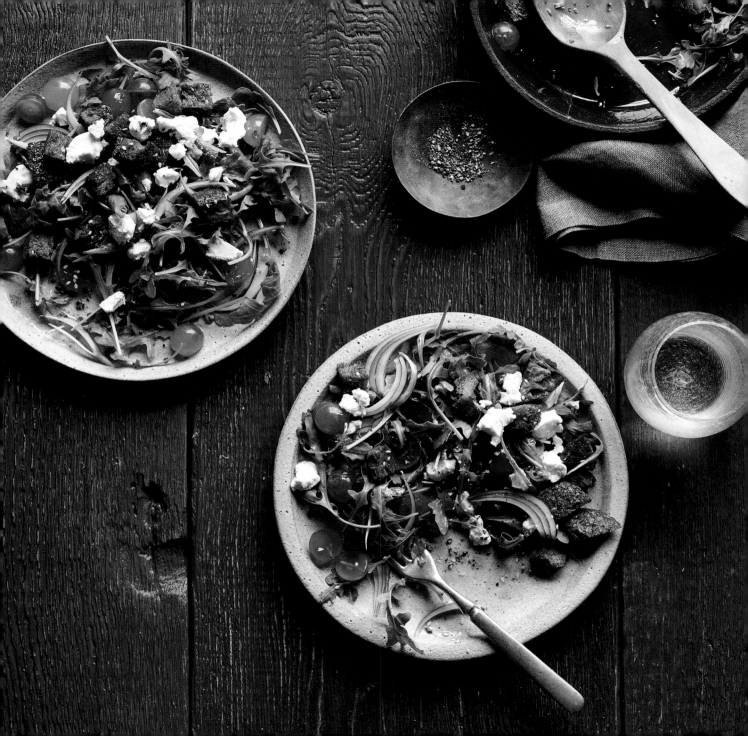

ARUGULA SALAD WITH GRAPES, GOAT CHEESE, AND ZA'ATAR CROUTONS

To mix things up, replace the grapes with fresh figs when they are in season.

PREP TIME: 10 MINUTES / TOTAL TIME: 20 MINUTES / SERVES 4

CROUTONS

- 2 slices whole wheat bread, cubed
- 2 teaspoons olive oil, divided
- 1 teaspoon za'atar

VINAIGRETTE

- 2 tablespoons olive oil
- 1 tablespoon red wine vinegar
- ½ teaspoon chopped fresh rosemary
- ¼ teaspoon kosher salt
- ⅛ teaspoon ground black pepper

SALAD

- 4 cups (4 ounces) baby arugula
- 1 cup grapes, halved
- ½ red onion, thinly sliced
- 2 ounces goat cheese, crumbled

1. *To make the croutons:* Toss the bread cubes with 1 teaspoon of the oil and the za'atar. In a medium skillet over medium heat, warm the remaining 1 teaspoon oil. Cook the bread cubes, stirring frequently, until browned and crispy, 8 to 10 minutes.

2. *To make the vinaigrette:* In a small bowl, whisk together the oil, vinegar, rosemary, salt, and pepper.

3. *To make the salad:* In a large bowl, toss the arugula, grapes, and onion with the vinaigrette. Top with the cheese and croutons.

Per serving: 204 calories, 6 g protein, 15 g carbohydrates, 8 g sugars, 14 g total fat, 4.5 g saturated fat, 2 g fiber, 283 mg sodium

ZA'ATAR

Italian, Spanish, and southern French cuisine are known for their liberal use of fresh herbs like rosemary, basil, parsley, and thyme. But in eastern Mediterranean countries like Israel, Lebanon, and Morocco, za'atar reigns supreme. This intensely aromatic spice blend is traditionally made with ground cumin, ground sumac, sesame seeds, and dried marjoram, oregano, and thyme. It's often rubbed onto grilled meats or sprinkled onto bread, but it's also a terrific way to add flavor to finished dishes. Try it as a garnish for hummus, savory yogurt bowls, or roasted vegetables.

MEDITERRANEAN NIÇOISE SALAD

This nod to the classic salad is a meal unto itself. All you need is a warm night and a glass of wine.

PREP TIME: 10 MINUTES / TOTAL TIME: 40 MINUTES / SERVES 4

¾ pound small red potatoes
  Kosher salt
2 eggs
¾ pound green beans, trimmed and halved
2 jars (6.7 ounces each) tuna fillets in olive oil (see note on page 110)
  Extra-virgin olive oil, if needed
1 small shallot, finely chopped
¼ cup white wine vinegar
1 teaspoon Dijon mustard
1 teaspoon chopped fresh thyme
  Ground black pepper
1 large head butter lettuce, such as Boston or Bibb, torn into bite-size pieces
1 cup cherry tomatoes, halved
½ cucumber, coarsely chopped
⅓ cup Niçoise olives

1. In a medium saucepan, add the potatoes, enough cold water to cover, and a big pinch of the salt and bring to a boil. Cook until the potatoes are tender, about 15 minutes. Using a slotted spoon, remove the potatoes to a bowl and let sit until cool enough to handle. Bring the pot of water back to a boil.

2. Carefully add the eggs to the boiling water, reduce the heat to a simmer, and cook for 15 minutes. Meanwhile, set up a large bowl of ice water. With a slotted spoon transfer the eggs to the ice water and let sit until cool, about 15 minutes. Bring the water back to a boil. Peel and quarter the eggs. Slice the potatoes into ¼" to ½" slices.

(continued)

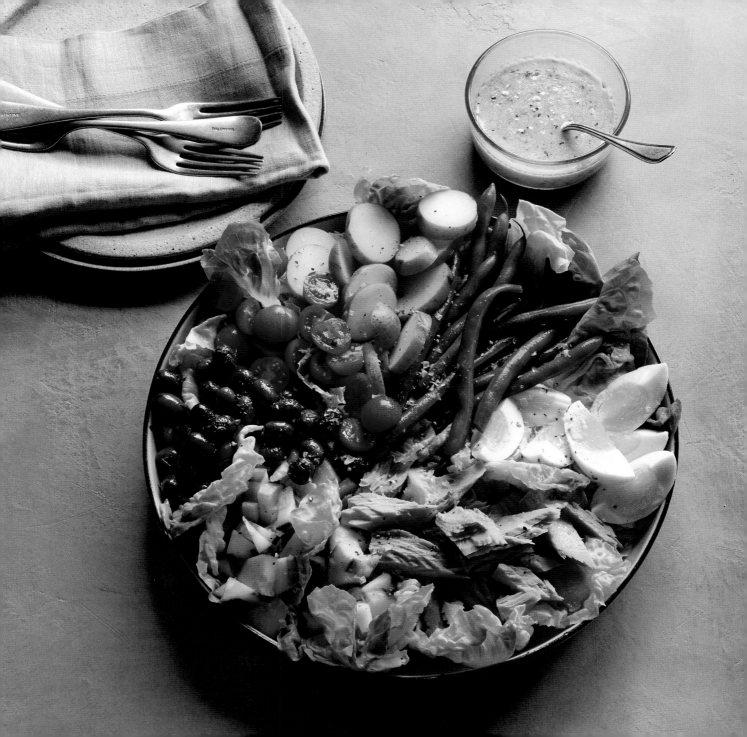

(continued from page 109)

3. Add the green beans to the boiling water. Cook until bright green and tender-crisp, about 3 minutes. Drain and add the beans to the ice water to stop cooking. Pat dry.

4. Drain the oil from the tuna into a small bowl. You will need 3 tablespoons; if there isn't enough, make up the difference with the extra-virgin olive oil. Whisk in the shallot, vinegar, mustard, thyme, and a pinch of the salt and pepper until completely combined.

5. On a large platter, spread out the lettuce and drizzle with a little of the dressing. Position the potato slices, hard-cooked egg quarters, green beans, tomatoes, cucumber, and olives over the lettuce in clusters with the flaked tuna in the center. Drizzle enough dressing to cover all of the salad and serve any remaining dressing on the side.

Per serving: 437 calories, 27 g protein, 31 g carbohydrates, 7 g sugars, 24 g total fat, 3 g saturated fat, 7 g fiber, 766 mg sodium

NOTE: For the tuna, we used Tonnino brand, which is 100 percent low-mercury yellowfin tuna.

WILD GREENS SALAD WITH FRESH HERBS

The types of wild greens (χόρτα, or *horta*) foraged on the island of Crete and in other Mediterranean countries differ from what's readily available in the United States. Here, we've used dandelion greens and chicory, both of which are slightly bitter, but any bitter green—beet, mustard, arugula—may be used. Cooking tames the bitterness, while the vinegar adds brightness. Vary the herbs to suit your taste. Serve this as they would in Crete, family-style.

PREP TIME: 10 MINUTES / TOTAL TIME: 30 MINUTES / SERVES 6 TO 8

¼ cup olive oil

2 pounds dandelion greens, tough stems removed and coarsely chopped

1 small bunch chicory, trimmed and coarsely chopped

1 cup chopped fresh flat-leaf parsley, divided

1 cup chopped fresh mint, divided

½ cup water

2 tablespoons red wine vinegar or apple cider vinegar

1 tablespoon fresh thyme, chopped

2 cloves garlic, minced

½ teaspoon kosher salt

½ teaspoon ground black pepper

¼ cup almonds or walnuts, coarsely chopped

2 tablespoons chopped fresh chives or scallion greens

1 tablespoon chopped fresh dill

1. In a large pot over medium heat, warm the oil. Add the greens, half of the parsley, half of the mint, the water, vinegar, thyme, garlic, salt, and pepper. Reduce the heat to a simmer and cook until the greens are very tender, about 20 minutes.

2. Meanwhile, in a small skillet over medium heat, toast the nuts until golden and fragrant, 5 to 8 minutes. Remove from the heat.

3. If serving immediately, stir the chives or scallion greens, dill, and the remaining parsley and mint into the pot. If serving as a cool or cold salad, allow to come to room temperature or refrigerate until cold before stirring in the fresh herbs. Top with the toasted nuts before serving.

Per serving: 190 calories, 6 g protein, 17 g carbohydrates, 1 g sugars, 13 g total fat, 2 g saturated fat, 7 g fiber, 279 mg sodium

SPINACH SALAD WITH POMEGRANATE, LENTILS, AND PISTACHIOS

Enjoy this sweet-savory salad as a light lunch with Whole Wheat Pitas (page 164) or as an accompaniment for grilled chicken or fish. Opt for French green lentils over standard brown lentils—they hold their shape better when cooked.

PREP TIME: 10 MINUTES / TOTAL TIME: 40 MINUTES / SERVES 4

1   tablespoon extra-virgin olive oil
1   shallot, finely chopped
1   small red chile pepper, such as a Fresno, finely chopped (wear plastic gloves when handling)
½   teaspoon ground cumin
¼   teaspoon ground coriander seeds
¼   teaspoon ground cinnamon
    Pinch of kosher salt
1   cup French green lentils, rinsed
3   cups water
6   cups (6 ounces) baby spinach
½   cup pomegranate seeds
¼   cup chopped fresh cilantro
¼   cup chopped fresh flat-leaf parsley
¼   cup chopped pistachi os
2   tablespoons fresh lemon juice
1   teaspoon finely grated lemon peel
    Ground black pepper, to taste

1. In a medium saucepan over medium heat, warm the oil until shimmering. Cook the shallot and chile pepper, stirring, until the shallot is translucent, about 8 minutes. Stir in the cumin, coriander, cinnamon, and salt until fragrant, about 1 minute. Add the lentils and water and bring to a boil. Cover and reduce the heat to a simmer. Cook, stirring occasionally, until the lentils are completely tender and the liquid has been absorbed, about 30 minutes.

2. In a large bowl, toss the lentils with the spinach, pomegranate seeds, cilantro, parsley, pistachios, lemon juice, lemon peel, and pepper to taste.

Per serving: 279 calories, 15 g protein, 39 g carbohydrates, 4 g sugars, 7 g total fat, 1 g saturated fat, 10 g fiber, 198 mg sodium

POMEGRANATES

Like grapes, pomegranates' deep garnet color is a sign that the fruits are loaded with polyphenols like resveratrol and anthocyanins. These powerful antioxidant compounds can help your heart, but that's not all: Research suggests that they might also boast cancer-fighting properties.[1] Add pomegranate seeds to salads or pilafs, stir them into yogurt or ricotta cheese, or enjoy them as a snack with a handful of nuts. The sweet-tart flavor and crunchy texture is always a treat. Pomegranate seeds, or arils as they are also called, can be found in the produce section of most grocery stores. To seed a whole pomegranate, quarter and then submerge it in a large bowl of water. Under the water, use your fingers to pry out the individual arils, leaving behind the pith. Watch out for errant sprays of red juice!

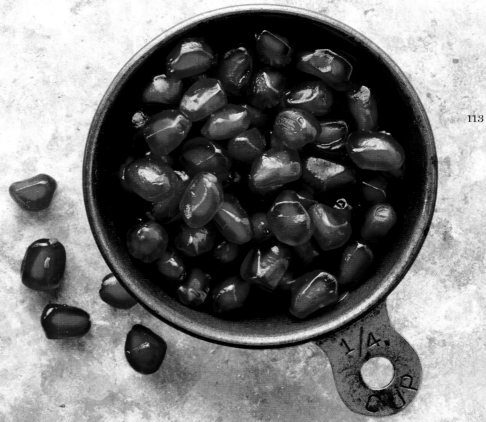

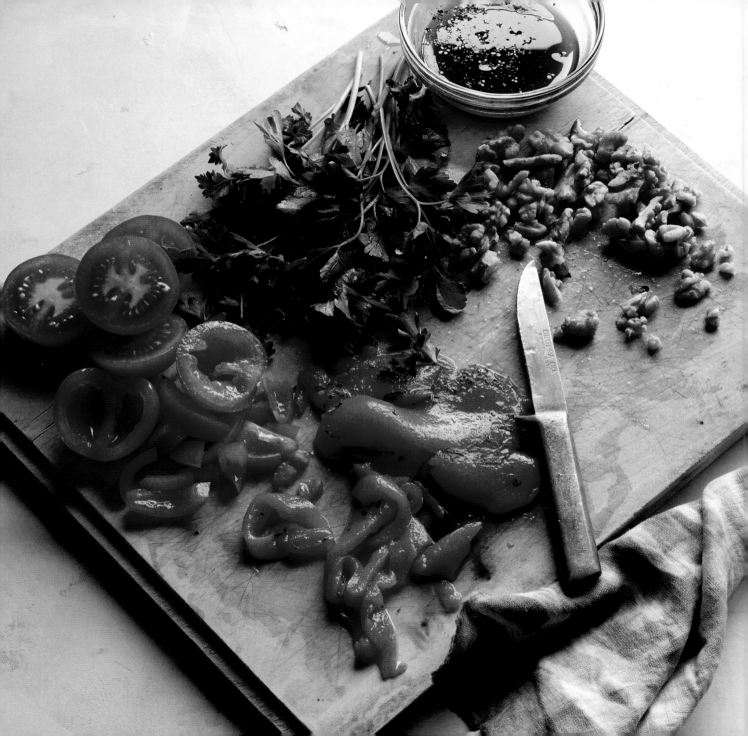

RED PEPPER, POMEGRANATE, AND WALNUT SALAD

This salad is terrific with Whole Wheat Pita (page 164) or piled on top of mixed greens.

PREP TIME: 5 MINUTES / TOTAL TIME: 45 MINUTES / SERVES 4

2 red bell peppers, halved and seeded
1 teaspoon plus 2 tablespoons olive oil
4 teaspoons pomegranate molasses, divided (see note)
2 teaspoons fresh lemon juice
¼ teaspoon kosher salt
⅛ teaspoon ground black pepper
4 plum tomatoes, halved, seeded, and chopped
¼ cup walnut halves, chopped
¼ cup chopped fresh flat-leaf parsley

1. Preheat the oven to 450°F.
2. Brush the bell peppers all over with 1 teaspoon of the oil and place cut side up on a large rimmed baking sheet. Drizzle 2 teaspoons of the pomegranate molasses in the cavities of the bell peppers. Roast the bell peppers until they have softened and the skins have charred, turning once during cooking, 30 to 40 minutes. Remove from the oven and cool to room temperature. Remove the skins and chop the peppers coarsely.
3. In a large bowl, whisk together the lemon juice, salt, black pepper, the remaining 2 tablespoons oil, and the remaining 2 teaspoons pomegranate molasses. Add the bell peppers, tomatoes, walnuts, and parsley and toss gently to combine. Serve at room temperature.

Per serving: 166 calories, 2 g protein, 11 g carbohydrates, 7 g sugars, 13 g total fat, 2 g saturated fat, 3 g fiber, 153 mg sodium

115

NOTE: Pomegranate molasses is available at well-stocked grocery stores and Middle Eastern markets. If you can't find it, substitute honey.

ROASTED CAULIFLOWER "STEAK" SALAD

Because this salad uses raw dandelion, look for younger, smaller greens found in the spring. If only bunches of larger dandelion greens are available (and you don't like the extra-bitter bite), opt for arugula instead. Use the leftover cauliflower florets to dip into Hummus (page 149) or for Arnabit (*Roasted Cauliflower*) with Spicy Tahini Sauce (page 177).

PREP TIME: 10 MINUTES / TOTAL TIME: 60 MINUTES / SERVES 4

2 tablespoons olive oil, divided
2 large heads cauliflower (about 3 pounds each), trimmed of outer leaves
2 teaspoons za'atar
1½ teaspoons kosher salt, divided
1¼ teaspoons ground black pepper, divided
1 teaspoon ground cumin
2 large carrots
8 ounces dandelion greens, tough stems removed
½ cup low-fat plain Greek yogurt
2 tablespoons tahini
2 tablespoons fresh lemon juice
1 tablespoon water
1 clove garlic, minced

1. Preheat the oven to 450°F. Brush a large baking sheet with some of the oil.

2. Place the cauliflower on a cutting board, stem side down. Cut down the middle, through the core and stem, and then cut two 1"-thick "steaks" from the middle. Repeat with the other cauliflower head. Set aside the remaining cauliflower for another use. Brush both sides of the steaks with the remaining oil and set on the baking sheet.

3. Combine the za'atar, 1 teaspoon of the salt, 1 teaspoon of the pepper, and the cumin. Sprinkle on the cauliflower steaks. Bake until the bottom is deeply golden, about 30 minutes. Flip and bake until tender, 10 to 15 minutes.

(continued)

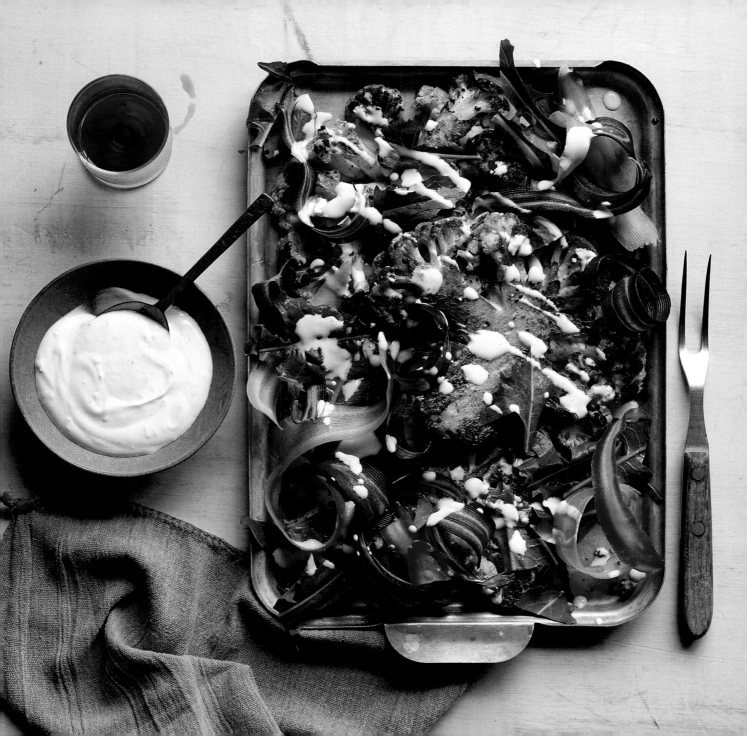

(continued from page 116)

4. Meanwhile, set the carrots on a cutting board and use a vegetable peeler to peel them into ribbons. Add to a large bowl with the dandelion greens.

5. In a small bowl, combine the yogurt, tahini, lemon juice, water, garlic, the remaining ½ teaspoon salt, and the remaining ¼ teaspoon pepper.

6. Dab 3 tablespoons of the dressing onto the carrot-dandelion mix. With a spoon or your hands, massage the dressing into the mix for 5 minutes.

7. Remove the steaks from the oven and transfer to individual plates. Drizzle each with 2 tablespoons of the dressing and top with 1 cup of the salad.

Per serving: 214 calories, 9 g protein, 21 g carbohydrates, 8 g sugars, 12 g total fat, 2 g saturated fat, 7 g fiber, 849 mg sodium

NOTE: Grilled chicken, shrimp, or lamb would make a lovely accompaniment to this salad. To keep it vegetarian, add 1 can drained-and-rinsed chickpeas or leftover cauliflower from the Roasted Cauliflower "Steak" Salad (page 116).

FATTOUSH
(LEBANESE PITA SALAD)

This Lebanese salad is truly out of this world. Be sure to use stale pita—save those fresh ones for sandwiches, such as the Baked Falafel with Tzatziki Sauce (page 134). This recipe calls for ground sumac, which is widely used in Mediterranean cooking and available in Middle Eastern markets and well-stocked supermarkets. If you can't find it, use za'atar.

PREP TIME: 10 MINUTES / TOTAL TIME: 20 MINUTES / SERVES 4 TO 6

2   Whole Wheat Pitas (page 164)
3   tablespoons extra-virgin olive oil, divided
½   teaspoon kosher salt, divided
1   head romaine lettuce, chopped into bite-size pieces
1   pint cherry or grape tomatoes, halved
1   English cucumber, chopped
1   small red onion, sliced, or 5 scallions, sliced
⅓   cup coarsely chopped fresh cilantro
⅓   cup coarsely chopped fresh mint
⅓   cup coarsely chopped fresh flat-leaf parsley
2   tablespoons fresh lemon juice
2   cloves garlic, minced
¾   teaspoon ground sumac

1. Brush the pitas with 1 teaspoon of the oil. Sprinkle with ¼ teaspoon of the salt. Toast until golden and crisp on both sides, either on a baking sheet in a 400°F oven for 5 to 10 minutes or in a toaster oven. Break into bite-size pieces and set aside.

2. In a large bowl, combine the lettuce, tomatoes, cucumber, onion or scallions, cilantro, mint, and parsley.

3. In a small bowl or jar with a lid, combine the lemon juice, garlic, sumac, the remaining oil, and the remaining ¼ teaspoon salt. Whisk together, or shake vigorously with the lid on, until emulsified. Pour over the vegetables and toss. Add the pita bits and toss again. Serve immediately.

Per serving: 246 calories, 7 g protein, 32 g carbohydrates, 6 g sugars, 12 g total fat, 1.5 g saturated fat, 8 g fiber, 444 mg sodium

119

BEETS WITH GOAT CHEESE AND CHERMOULA

Chermoula is a marinade or sauce used in many Mediterranean countries, including Algeria, Morocco, and Tunisia. There are a lot of regional variations—you can include (or substitute) onion, ground black pepper, saffron, or ground chile pepper in your version.

PREP TIME: 10 MINUTES / TOTAL TIME: 50 MINUTES / SERVES 4

6 beets, trimmed

CHERMOULA

1	cup fresh cilantro leaves
1	cup fresh flat-leaf parsley leaves
¼	cup fresh lemon juice
3	cloves garlic, minced
2	teaspoons ground cumin
1	teaspoon smoked paprika
½	teaspoon kosher salt
¼	teaspoon chili powder (optional)
¼	cup extra-virgin olive oil
2	ounces goat cheese, crumbled

1. Preheat the oven to 400°F.

2. Wrap the beets in a piece of foil and place on a baking sheet. Roast until the beets are tender enough to be pierced with a fork, 30 to 40 minutes. When cool enough to handle, remove the skins and slice the beets into ¼" rounds. Arrange the beet slices on a large serving platter.

3. *To make the chermoula:* In a food processor, pulse the cilantro, parsley, lemon juice, garlic, cumin, paprika, salt, and chili powder (if using) until the herbs are just coarsely chopped and the ingredients are combined. Stir in the oil.

4. To serve, dollop the chermoula over the beets and scatter the cheese on top.

Per serving: 249 calories, 6 g protein, 15 g carbohydrates, 9 g sugars, 19 g total fat, 5 g saturated fat, 5 g fiber, 472 mg sodium

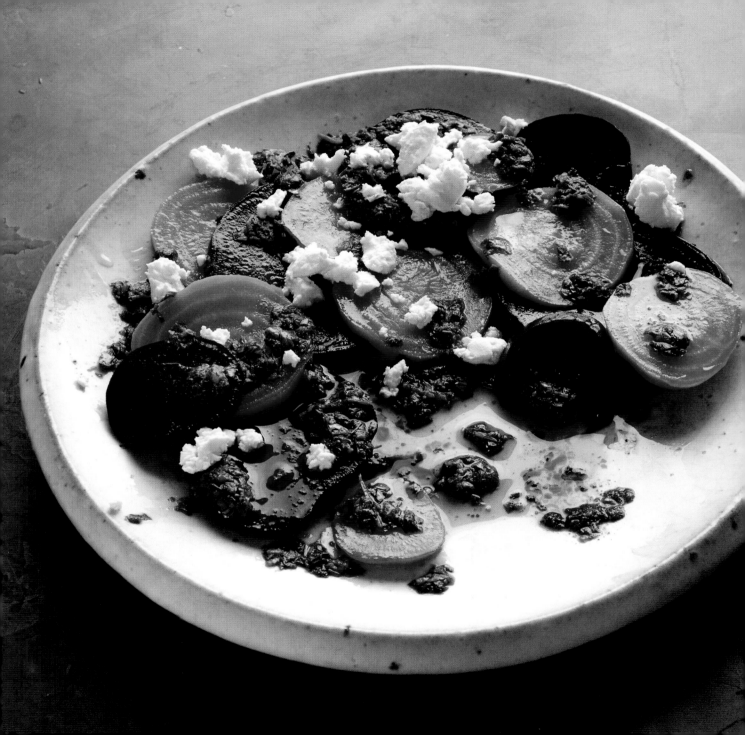

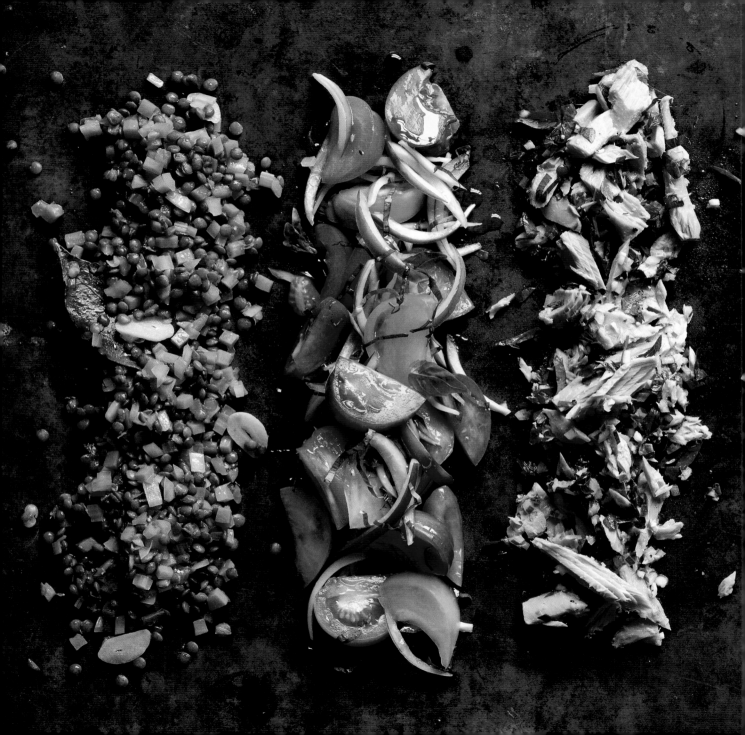

MEZE PLATE— TUNA SALAD, LENTIL SALAD, TOMATO SALAD

Are you familiar with Spanish tapas? Then you already know a bit about meze, the eastern Mediterranean's version of small-plate meals that are perfect for no-fuss entertaining. Similar to tapas, meze often includes a collection of appetizer-style dishes (called *mezedhes*) such as pita, dips, salads, cheeses, grilled fish, and meatballs like Baked Turkey Kibbeh (page 188).

TUNA SALAD // PREP TIME: 5 MINUTES / TOTAL TIME: 15 MINUTES / SERVES 4

LENTIL SALAD // PREP TIME: 10 MINUTES / TOTAL TIME: 90 MINUTES / SERVES 4

TOMATO SALAD // PREP TIME: 5 MINUTES / TOTAL TIME: 10 MINUTES / SERVES 4

TUNA SALAD

¼ cup fresh lemon juice
¼ red onion, finely chopped
1 clove garlic, minced
2 jars (6.7 ounces each) tuna fillets in oil, drained (see note on page 110)
¼ cup chopped fresh flat-leaf parsley
Kosher salt and ground black pepper, to taste

In a medium bowl, combine the lemon juice, onion, and garlic and let sit to meld for 5 minutes. Flake in the tuna and toss in the dressing with the parsley. Season to taste with the salt and pepper.

Per serving: 141 calories, 19 g protein, 2 g carbohydrates, 1 g sugars, 6 g total fat, 1 g saturated fat, 0 g fiber, 403 mg sodium

TOMATO SALAD

4 large ripe tomatoes, cut into 1" wedges
¼ small red onion, thinly sliced
4 large leaves basil, thinly sliced
1 tablespoon extra-virgin olive oil
Kosher salt and ground black pepper, to taste

In a medium bowl, toss the tomatoes, onion, basil, and oil together. Season to taste with the salt and pepper.

Per serving: 57 calories, 1 g protein, 6 g carbohydrates, 4 g sugars, 4 g total fat, 0.5 g saturated fat, 2 g fiber, 127 mg sodium

(continued)

LENTILS

Like all beans and legumes, lentils aren't just good for your waistline. They can also help your heart. Half a cup of cooked lentils serves up 8 grams of fiber, which is known to help lower levels of LDL (bad) cholesterol. They are also rich in potassium and magnesium, two minerals that play an important role in maintaining healthy blood pressure. Try brown lentils for soups—their texture softens during cooking, thickening the broth. French green lentils are ideal for salads since they stay firm even after cooking.

(continued from page 123)

LENTIL SALAD

½   cup brown or French green lentils, rinsed
1   small onion, diced
1   carrot, diced
1   small rib celery, diced
2   cloves garlic
1   bay leaf
2   tablespoons extra-virgin olive oil
2   tablespoons sherry vinegar
2   scallions, thinly sliced
    Kosher salt and ground black pepper, to taste

In a small saucepan with enough water to cover over medium-high heat, bring the lentils, onion, carrot, celery, garlic, and bay leaf to a boil. Reduce the heat to a simmer and cook until the lentils are tender, about 30 minutes. Let the lentils cool completely in their liquid and drain. Remove and discard the garlic and bay leaf. In a medium bowl, toss the lentils with the oil, vinegar, and scallions. Season to taste with the salt and pepper.

Per serving: 158 calories, 6 g protein, 18 g carbohydrates, 2 g sugars, 8 g total fat, 1 g saturated fat, 5 g fiber, 263 mg sodium

PEAR-FENNEL SALAD WITH POMEGRANATE

To get the ideal thinness on the pear and fennel for this delicate salad, you will need to use a mandoline. But if you don't have one, simply slice carefully with a sharp knife. Turn this salad into a meal by topping it with grilled salmon or chicken.

PREP TIME: I5 MINUTES / TOTAL TIME: 20 MINUTES / SERVES 6

DRESSING

- 2 tablespoons red wine vinegar
- 1½ tablespoons pomegranate molasses (see note on page II5)
- 2 teaspoons finely chopped shallot
- ½ teaspoon Dijon mustard
- ½ teaspoon kosher salt
- ¼ teaspoon ground black pepper
- ¼ cup extra-virgin olive oil

SALAD

- ¼ cup walnuts, coarsely chopped, or pine nuts
- 2 red pears, halved, cored, and very thinly sliced
- I bulb fennel, halved, cored, and very thinly sliced, fronds reserved
- I tablespoon fresh lemon juice
- 4 cups (4 ounces) baby arugula
- ½ cup pomegranate seeds
- ⅓ cup crumbled feta cheese or shaved Parmigiano-Reggiano cheese

1. *To make the dressing:* In a small bowl or jar with a lid, combine the vinegar, pomegranate molasses, shallot, mustard, salt, and pepper. Add the oil and whisk until emulsified (or cap the jar and shake vigorously). Set aside.

2. *To make the salad:* In a small skillet over medium heat, toast the nuts until golden and fragrant, 4 to 5 minutes. Remove from the skillet to cool.

3. In a large bowl, combine the pears and fennel. Sprinkle with the lemon juice and toss gently.

4. Add the arugula and toss again to evenly distribute. Pour over 3 to 4 tablespoons of the dressing, just enough to moisten the arugula, and toss. Add the pomegranate seeds, cheese, and nuts and toss again. Add more dressing, if necessary, or store remainder in the refrigerator for up to 1 week. Serve the salad topped with the reserved fennel fronds.

Per serving: 165 calories, 3 g protein, 18 g carbohydrates, 10 g sugars, 10 g total fat, 2.5 g saturated fat, 4 g fiber, 215 mg sodium

125

PANZANELLA
(TUSCAN BREAD AND TOMATOES SALAD)

Traditionally, Italians make panzanella to use up day-old bread. But grilling fresh bread with a touch of olive oil yields even tastier results.

PREP TIME: 10 MINUTES / TOTAL TIME: 30 MINUTES / SERVES 6

4 ounces sourdough bread, cut into I" slices (see note)
3 tablespoons extra-virgin olive oil, divided
2 tablespoons red wine vinegar
2 cloves garlic, mashed to a paste
1 teaspoon finely chopped fresh oregano or ½ teaspoon dried
1 teaspoon fresh thyme leaves
½ teaspoon Dijon mustard
Pinch of kosher salt
Few grinds of ground black pepper
2 pounds ripe tomatoes (mixed colors)
6 ounces fresh mozzarella pearls
1 cucumber, cut into ½"-thick half-moons
1 small red onion, thinly sliced
1 cup (1ounce) baby arugula
½ cup torn fresh basil

1. Coat a grill rack or grill pan with olive oil and prepare to medium-high heat.

2. Brush 1 tablespoon of the oil all over the bread slices. Grill the bread on both sides until grill marks appear, about 2 minutes per side. Cut the bread into 1" cubes.

3. In a large bowl, whisk together the vinegar, garlic, oregano, thyme, mustard, salt, pepper, and the remaining 2 tablespoons oil until emulsified.

4. Add the bread, tomatoes, mozzarella, cucumber, onion, arugula, and basil. Toss to combine and let sit for 10 minutes to soak up the flavors.

Per serving: 219 calories, 10 g protein, 19 g carbohydrates, 6 g sugars, 12 g total fat, 4 g saturated fat, 3 g fiber, 222 mg sodium

GRILLED HALLOUMI WITH MIXED GRILLED VEGETABLES

When cooked at a high temperature, Halloumi cheese turns crispy and caramelized on the outside. But unlike most cheeses, it holds it shape instead of melting.

PREP TIME: 15 MINUTES / TOTAL TIME: 45 MINUTES / SERVES 4

1   large eggplant, cut into ½"-thick slices
1   pound asparagus, trimmed
2   large red bell peppers, quartered and seeded
1   large red onion, cut into ½"-thick slices
6   ounces Halloumi cheese, cut into ½"-thick slices
2   large ears corn, shucked
4   tablespoons olive oil, divided
3   tablespoons balsamic vinegar
1   teaspoon finely chopped fresh rosemary
1   clove garlic, mashed to a paste
¼   teaspoon red-pepper flakes
    Pinch of kosher salt

1. Coat a grill rack or grill pan with olive oil and prepare to medium-high heat.

2. Brush the eggplant, asparagus, bell peppers, onion, cheese, and corn all over with 2 tablespoons of the oil. Transfer to the grill and cook until pronounced grill marks form on 2 sides and the vegetables are tender, about 10 minutes for the onion, bell peppers, and corn, about 6 minutes for the eggplant, and about 4 minutes for the cheese and asparagus.

3. Meanwhile, in a large bowl, whisk together the vinegar, rosemary, garlic, pepper flakes, salt, and the remaining 2 tablespoons oil.

4. Transfer the cheese and all the vegetables to a cutting board. Coarsely chop the onion, bell pepper, eggplant, and asparagus and add it to the bowl. Cut the cheese into bite-size pieces and add to the bowl. Cut the corn off the cob and transfer to the bowl. Toss and let sit for 5 minutes to meld the flavors.

Per serving: 373 calories, 15 g protein, 32 g carbohydrates, 16 g sugars, 29 g total fat, 11 g saturated fat, 9 g fiber, 912 mg sodium

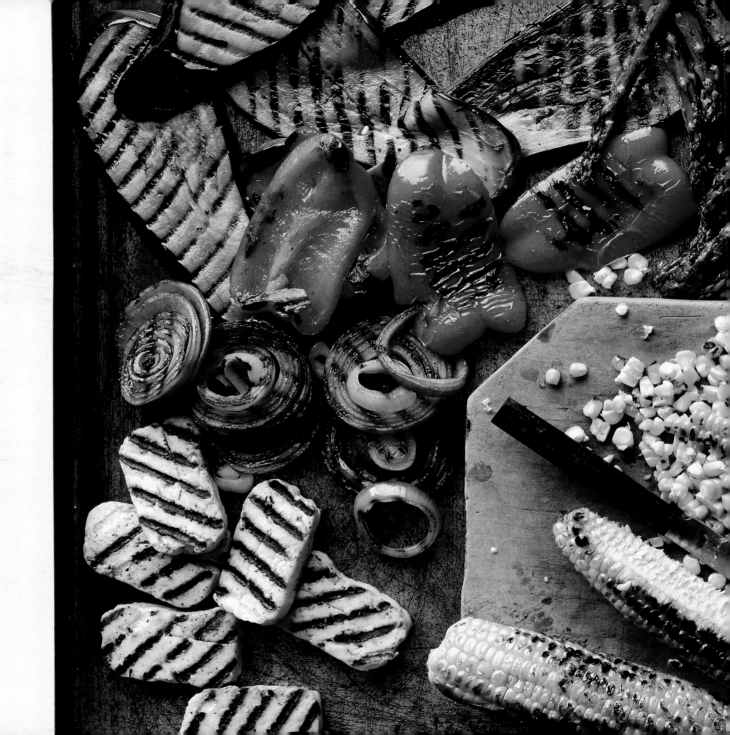

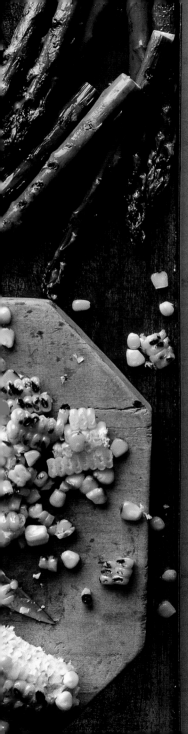

HALLOUMI

Feta isn't the only cheese you'll find at Greek tables. Also a staple, Halloumi is a semihard cheese made from goat's or sheep's milk. It has a higher melting point than most cheeses, so it holds up to grilling and pan-searing. And if you're still skeptical that Halloumi and other cheeses can be part of a healthy eating pattern, consider this: Consumption of moderate full-fat cheeses has been linked to a lower risk for heart disease[2] and stroke,[3] as well as a longer life span.[4] Though cheese is high in saturated fat, it's got some good stuff going for it, too. Namely, palmitoleate, an anti-inflammatory fatty acid that research suggests could help neutralize saturated fat's harmful effects.[5] And because cheese is a fermented food, it serves up probiotic bacteria that could boost your gut health—and even help rev your metabolism.

CALAMARI SALAD

Light and refreshing, calamari salad is a staple in coastal Italian regions. Take care not to cook the squid for too long, as it can quickly turn tough.

PREP TIME: 15 MINUTES / TOTAL TIME: 30 MINUTES / SERVES 4

1 pound cleaned squid with tentacles, bodies cut into ½"-thick rings
6 tablespoons olive oil
Juice of 1 lime
1 clove garlic, minced
1 teaspoon kosher salt
½ teaspoon ground black pepper
½ cup chopped fresh cilantro
½ cup chopped fresh mint
2 scallions, thinly sliced
1 rib celery, chopped
1 jalapeño chile pepper, seeded and minced (optional), wear plastic gloves when handling

1. Bring a large pot of salted water to a boil and have a bowl of ice water ready.
2. Add the squid to the boiling water and cook until just opaque, 40 to 60 seconds. Remove the squid with a slotted spoon and immediately transfer to the ice water to stop cooking. Once cooled, drain the squid and pat dry.
3. In a large serving bowl, whisk together the oil, lime juice, garlic, salt, and black pepper. Stir in the cilantro, mint, scallions, celery, chile pepper (if using), and squid and let stand for 15 minutes to allow the flavors to mingle.

Per serving: 278 calories, 18 g protein, 7 g carbohydrates, 1 g sugars, 20 g total fat, 3 g saturated fat, 1 g fiber, 643 mg sodium

130

KIDNEY BEAN PEASANT SALAD

This humble salad is hearty enough to stand on its own for dinner or a great accompaniment to roast chicken, fish, or lamb.

PREP TIME: 10 MINUTES / TOTAL TIME: 45 MINUTES / SERVES 8

1   large shallot, very thinly sliced
3   tablespoons fresh lemon juice or white wine vinegar
2   tablespoons chopped fresh mint
2   tablespoons chopped fresh flat-leaf parsley
1   teaspoon mustard powder
1   teaspoon ground sumac
½   teaspoon kosher salt
½   teaspoon ground black pepper
⅓   cup extra-virgin olive oil
2   cans (15 ounces each) red kidney beans, drained and rinsed (see note on page 80)
2   cans (15 ounces each) cannellini beans, drained and rinsed (see note on page 80)
1   English cucumber, chopped
1   large tomato, chopped

1. In a large bowl, whisk together the shallot, lemon juice, mint, parsley, mustard, sumac, salt, and pepper. Stream in the oil, whisking, until emulsified.

2. Add the beans, cucumber, and tomato and lightly toss to coat. Set aside, refrigerated or at room temperature, for 30 minutes for the flavors to blend. Serve chilled or at room temperature.

131

Per serving: 215 calories, 9 g protein, 25 g carbohydrates, 4 g sugars, 9 g total fat, 1 g saturated fat, 8 g fiber, 505 mg sodium

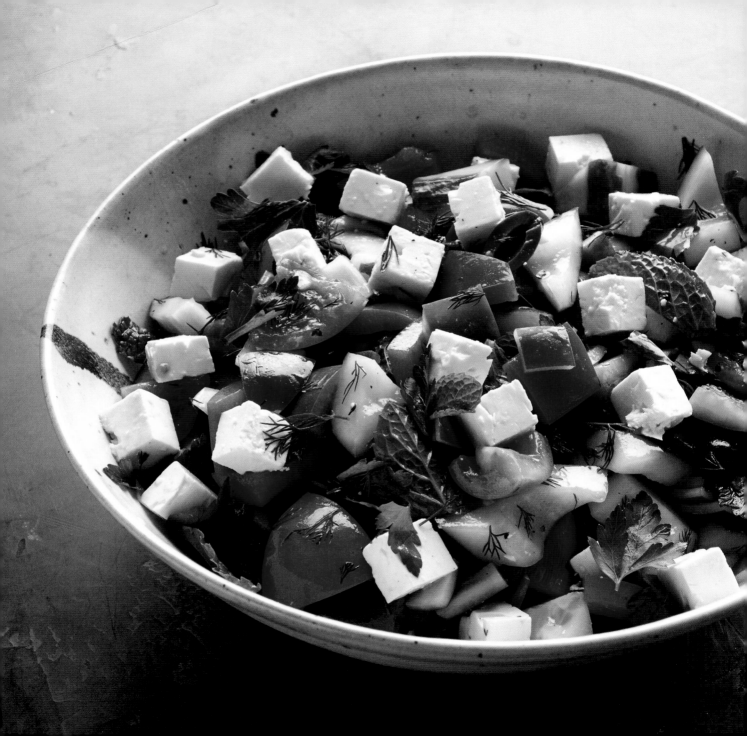

TURKISH SHEPHERD'S SALAD

Every Turkish cook has their own version of this refreshing summer salad. Enjoy it for lunch with crusty whole grain bread or Whole Wheat Pitas (page 164).

PREP TIME: 15 MINUTES / TOTAL TIME: 15 MINUTES / SERVES 6

¼ cup extra-virgin olive oil
2 tablespoons apple cider vinegar
2 tablespoons lemon juice
½ teaspoon kosher salt
¼ teaspoon ground black pepper
3 plum tomatoes, seeded and chopped
2 cucumbers, seeded and chopped
1 red bell pepper, seeded and chopped
1 green bell pepper, seeded and chopped
1 small red onion, chopped
⅓ cup pitted black olives (such as kalamata), halved
½ cup chopped fresh flat-leaf parsley
¼ cup chopped fresh mint
¼ cup chopped fresh dill
6 ounces feta cheese, cubed

1. In a small bowl, whisk together the oil, vinegar, lemon juice, salt, and black pepper.
2. In a large serving bowl, combine the tomatoes, cucumber, bell peppers, onion, olives, parsley, mint, and dill. Pour the dressing over the salad, toss gently, and sprinkle with the cheese.

Per serving: 238 calories, 6 g protein, 10 g carbohydrates, 5 g sugars, 20 g total fat, 6 g saturated fat, 2 g fiber, 806 mg sodium

133

BAKED FALAFEL WITH TZATZIKI SAUCE

Traditional falafel recipes call for dried chickpeas and deep-frying. This one uses canned chickpeas and bakes the falafel balls in the oven. The result is quicker and less messy—but just as delicious.

PREP TIME: 15 MINUTES / TOTAL TIME: 30 MINUTES / SERVES 8 (3 FALAFEL AND ABOUT ⅓ CUP TZATZIKI PER SERVING)

FALAFEL

- 2 tablespoons olive oil, divided
- 2 cans (15 ounces each) chickpeas, drained and rinsed (see note on page 80)
- 1 yellow onion, coarsely chopped
- 1 cup fresh flat-leaf parsley leaves or cilantro leaves
- 1 tablespoon lemon juice
- 2 cloves garlic
- ½ teaspoon ground cumin
- ¼ teaspoon kosher salt
- ¼ teaspoon ground black pepper
- ½ cup whole wheat bread crumbs
- ½ teaspoon baking powder

TZATZIKI SAUCE

- 1½ cups low-fat plain Greek yogurt
- 1 cucumber, diced
- 2 tablespoons finely chopped fresh dill
- 2 tablespoons finely chopped fresh mint
- 2 tablespoons lemon juice
- 1 clove garlic, minced
- ½ teaspoon kosher salt
- ¼ teaspoon ground black pepper
- ¼ teaspoon ground cumin

- 4 Whole Wheat Pitas (page 164), halved and split
- 1 large tomato, chopped
- ¼ cup pitted kalamata olives, halved

134

1. *To make the falafel:* Preheat the oven to 375°F. Coat a large baking sheet with 1 tablespoon of the oil.

2. In a food processor, pulse the chickpeas until broken up. Add the onion, parsley or cilantro, lemon juice, garlic, cumin, salt, and pepper. Pulse until pasty but not pureed. Pulse in the bread crumbs and baking powder until the mixture firms up.

3. Form 24 golf ball–size balls of the chickpea mix and place on the baking sheet. Gently press to flatten slightly. Brush the tops with the remaining 1 tablespoon oil. Bake until golden, 10 to 15 minutes.

4. *To make the tzatziki:* Meanwhile, in a medium bowl, combine the yogurt, cucumber, dill, mint, lemon juice, garlic, salt, pepper, and cumin.

5. To serve, put 3 falafel in each pita half, drizzle with ⅓ cup of the tzatziki, and top with the tomato and olives.

Per serving: 279 calories, 12 g protein, 39 g carbohydrates, 4 g sugars, 9 g total fat, 2 g saturated fat, 7 g fiber, 811 mg sodium

LEBANESE GARLIC CHICKEN FLATBREADS

You may be tempted to skip the long marinating time here, but trust us when we say that it will be worth the wait! And the cucumbers will add a fresh crunch!

PREP TIME: 5 MINUTES / TOTAL TIME: 25 MINUTES PLUS MARINATING TIME / SERVES 6

8	cloves garlic
½	teaspoon kosher salt
¼	cup olive oil
2	tablespoons fresh lemon juice
½	teaspoon ground sumac
1	pound boneless, skinless chicken thighs
1	cup thinly sliced cucumber
6	whole wheat flatbreads

1. In a medium bowl, muddle the garlic and salt together using the end of a wooden spoon, or use a mortar and pestle if you have one. Add the oil, lemon juice, and sumac and stir into a thick paste.

2. Place the chicken thighs in a gallon-size resealable plastic bag and pour the garlic mixture over the top. Massage the marinade into the chicken and place in the fridge for 6 hours or overnight.

3. Coat a grill rack or grill pan with olive oil and prepare to medium-high heat.

4. Remove the chicken from the marinade and discard the marinade. Grill the chicken until grill marks form and a thermometer inserted in the thickest part reaches 165°F, about 10 minutes per side.

5. Slice the chicken into bite-size pieces and distribute, along with the cucumber slices, among 6 flatbreads. Roll the flatbreads around the chicken and serve.

Per serving: 407 calories, 37 g protein, 37 g carbohydrates, 0 g sugars, 13 g total fat, 2 g saturated fat, 5 g fiber, 154 mg sodium

136

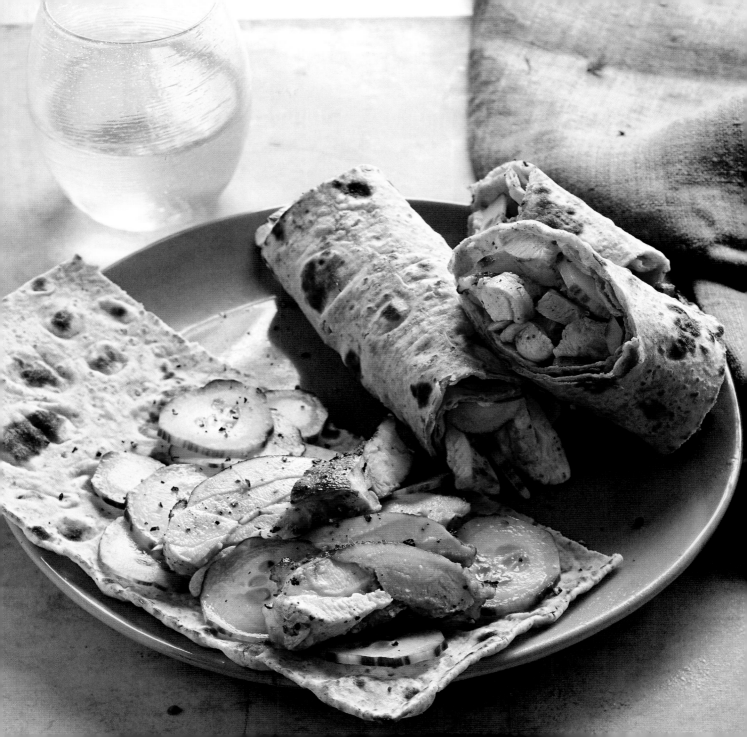

GARLIC

You might not want to put a garlic-heavy dish on the menu for a romantic meal, but these highly pungent, fragrant cloves are still good for the heart. The organosulfur compounds that give garlic its unmistakable flavor and aroma have been found to keep blood platelets from sticking together and prevent harmful clots from forming. Garlic also helps relax blood vessels and fights atherosclerosis—the hardening of arteries—and could even help keep your cholesterol in check. In a *Nutrition Reviews* analysis of nearly 40 studies, researchers concluded that regular garlic consumption could lower total cholesterol by up to 9 points—and reduce the risk of problems like heart attacks and strokes by as much as 38 percent.[6] Pretty impressive for a simple flavor enhancer! If garlic tends to leave you gassy or give you vampire breath, try the Italian custom of chewing fennel seeds after your meal. Essential oils in the seeds can enhance digestion, as well as neutralize the odor of your garlicky meal. Not a fan of fennel? Try munching on a sprig of fresh parsley or mint instead.

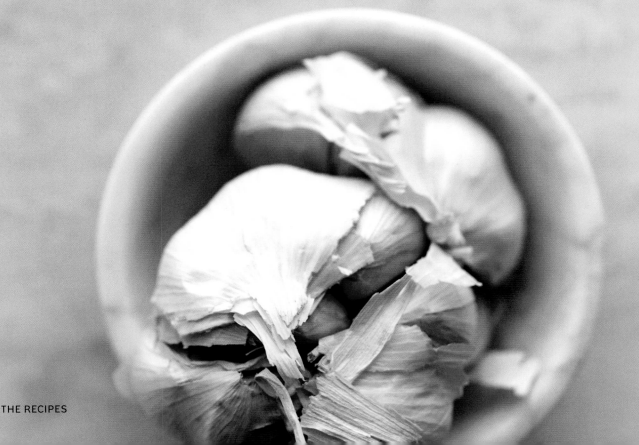

GREEK SALAD PITAS WITH TAPENADE SPREAD

All the flavors of a classic Greek salad—packed into a portable pita that's easy to pack for lunch or picnics.

PREP TIME: 15 MINUTES / TOTAL TIME: 15 MINUTES / SERVES 4

TAPENADE

½ cup pitted kalamata olives
2 tablespoons drained capers
2 tablespoons coarsely chopped fresh flat-leaf parsley
2 tablespoons fresh oregano
2 teaspoons extra-virgin olive oil
Ground black pepper, to taste

4 Whole Wheat Pitas (page 164), halved and split
1 head romaine lettuce, chopped
4 plum tomatoes, sliced into rounds
½ red onion, thinly sliced
2 ounces feta cheese, crumbled

1. *To make the tapenade:* Using a food processor or a knife, pulse or chop the olives, capers, parsley, and oregano until a chunky paste forms. Transfer to a small bowl and stir in the oil and season to taste with the pepper.

2. To assemble, spread 1 tablespoon of the tapenade inside each pita half. Divide the lettuce, tomato, onion, and cheese evenly among the halves.

139

Per serving: 309 calories, 11 g protein, 47 g carbohydrates, 5 g sugars, 11 g total fat, 3.5 g saturated fat, 9 g fiber, 937 mg sodium

TURKEY BURGERS WITH FETA AND DILL

The surprise of these burgers is that the dill and feta cheese are on the inside. Feel free to top with some tzatziki sauce (page 134), or try Mixed-Olive Tapenade (page 163).

PREP TIME: 5 MINUTES / TOTAL TIME: 20 MINUTES / SERVES 4

I   pound ground turkey breast
I   small red onion, ½ finely chopped, ½ sliced
½   cup crumbled feta cheese
¼   cup chopped fresh dill
I   clove garlic, minced
½   teaspoon kosher salt
¼   teaspoon ground black pepper
4   whole grain hamburger rolls or Whole Wheat Pitas (page 164)
4   thick slices tomato
4   leaves lettuce

1. Coat a grill rack or grill pan with olive oil and prepare to medium-high heat.

2. In a large bowl, use your hands to combine the turkey, chopped onion, cheese, dill, garlic, salt, and pepper. Do not overmix. Divide into 4 patties, 4" in diameter.

3. Grill the patties, covered, until a thermometer inserted in the center registers 165°F, 5 to 6 minutes per side.

4. Serve each patty on a roll or pita with the sliced onion, 1 slice of the tomato, and 1 leaf of the lettuce.

Per serving (with whole grain hamburger rolls): 305 calories, 35 g protein, 26 g carbohydrates, 5 g sugars, 7 g total fat, 3 g saturated fat, 3 g fiber, 708 mg sodium

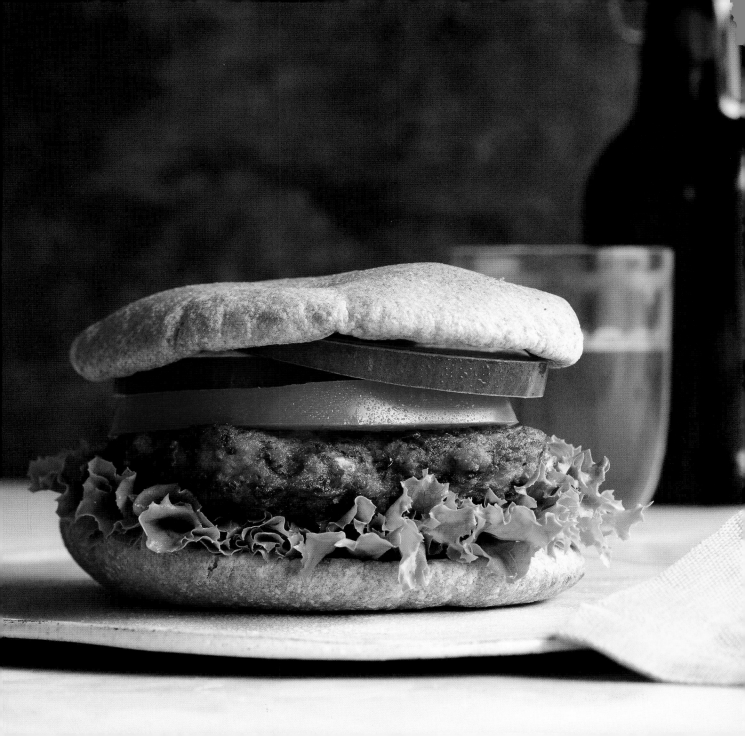

Chapter 6
Snacks and Sides

We'll be upfront here: Snacks aren't nearly as popular in the Mediterranean as they are here at home. Eating in between meals—especially on the go—isn't much a part of the culture. And it isn't even all that necessary: Since most Mediterranean eaters have their main meal midday, snacking in the morning might spoil their appetite. And if you ate a slow multicourse lunch, your stomach probably isn't grumbling at 3:30 p.m.

That's not to say that Mediterranean eaters *never* snack. In countries like Spain or Italy, for instance, some folks will sit down to a small late-afternoon nosh to tide them over until dinner (which might not be until 9:00 or 10:00 p.m.). And snacks can certainly have a place in a Mediterranean-style diet here at home, too. Well-timed nibbles can help you avoid getting overly hungry, so you're able to actually enjoy your meals at a leisurely pace. After all, it's tough to resist scarfing down your lunch or dinner when you're starving!

The key is sticking to simple, satisfying snacks, like the ones found in this chapter, instead of reaching for highly processed foods. Listening to your appetite matters, too, since it can help you avoid snacking mindlessly. These simple tips can help.

• **PLAN YOUR SNACKS.** When Mediterranean eaters *do* have a bite, it tends to be intentional. Rather than grabbing a snack thoughtlessly, think about the times you tend to get hungriest, and make it a point to have your snacks then. Planning ahead can help you avoid mindless snacking, plus it makes your snack feel more like a ritual that you can look forward to.

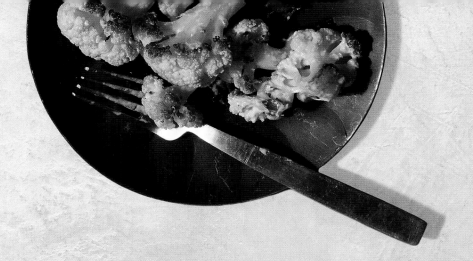

• **ONLY SNACK WHEN YOU'RE HUNGRY.**
There's no rule saying you have to eat just because of what the clock says. When your usual snack time rolls around, check in with your stomach before you begin nibbling. If you're truly hungry, go ahead and eat something. But if you aren't, hold off on eating until your next meal. You don't *have* to snack.

• **EAT REAL FOOD.** Mediterranean-style snacks look a lot like Mediterranean-style meals or the components of Mediterranean meals: They're made with real, wholesome ingredients, and they tend not to come in a box or bag. Instead of chips or a granola bar, reach for nuts, veggies with hummus, yogurt with fresh fruit, or a cube or two of cheese. Another idea: Prep simple side dishes, like the veggie sides in this chapter, ahead of time, and have small helpings as snacks throughout the week.

• **LOOK TO YOUR LEFTOVERS.** There's no rule that says snacks need to consist of, well, snack foods. Leftovers from a recent meal—like a wedge of frittata or a small cup of soup or bean salad—are always an option!

143

Recipes

144

145

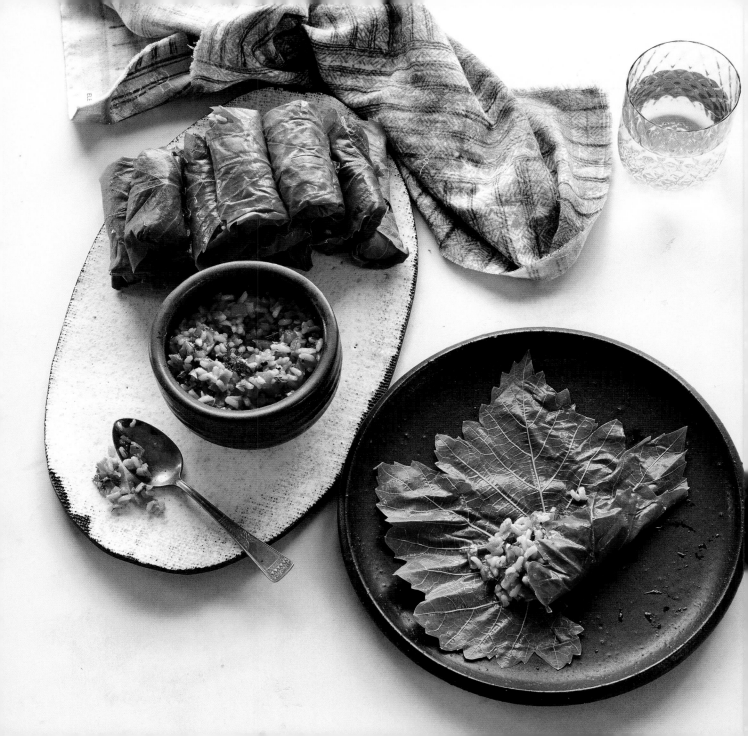

VEGETARIAN DOLMADES (STUFFED GRAPE LEAVES)

Pickled grape leaves are sold online or at Mediterranean markets. They also sell grape leaves in water; depending on the brand, they may need additional boiling to soften enough to roll.

PREP TIME: 15 MINUTES / TOTAL TIME: 2 HOURS 20 MINUTES / SERVES ABOUT 20 (3 PER SERVING)

½   cup olive oil, divided
1   onion, finely chopped
1½ cups quick-cooking brown rice
3   cloves garlic, minced
¾   cup low-sodium vegetable broth
2   tomatoes, finely chopped
¼   cup chopped fresh dill
¼   cup chopped fresh flat-leaf parsley
6   tablespoons fresh lemon juice, divided
1   tablespoon grated lemon peel
    Kosher salt and ground black pepper, to taste
1   jar (16 ounces) pickled grape leaves
    (about 70 leaves)

1. In a medium saucepan over medium heat, warm 3 tablespoons of the oil until shimmering. Cook the onion, stirring until translucent, about 5 minutes. Stir in the rice and garlic and cook, stirring, until the garlic is fragrant and the rice is coated in oil and slightly toasted, about 2 minutes. Add the broth and cook until the rice is only half cooked, about 5 minutes.

2. Remove the rice from the heat and stir in the tomatoes, dill, parsley, 2 tablespoons of the lemon juice, and the lemon peel. Season to taste with the salt and pepper.

3. Remove the grape leaves from the jar, rinse under cold water, and squeeze gently. Spread a leaf shiny side down and place 1 tablespoon of the filling in the center. Fold the bottom of the leaf (where the stem was) over the filling, fold the 2 sides into the center, and then roll into a cylinder. Repeat with the remaining filling

147

(continued)

(continued from page 147)

148

and leaves, setting aside any broken or unusable leaves. You may have leftover filling; use it in stuffed peppers, or freeze it for your next time making dolmades.

4. Cover the bottom of a large pot with the broken grape leaves. If you don't have enough, place a layer of wooden skewers down. You don't want the dolmades touching the bottom of the pot (they make break or burn). Arrange the dolmades in a single layer, tightly against each other, with the seam side down. When the first layer is complete, add another in the same way, until all the dolmades are in.

5. Drizzle the remaining 5 tablespoons oil over all the dolmades. Place a plate over the dolmades with a weight on top (such as a jar of water or a smaller pot) to keep it from floating up. Add enough water to cover the plate by 1". Bring to a simmer, reduce the heat to low, and cook for 40 minutes.

6. Remove the weight and plate and pour the remaining $\frac{1}{4}$ cup lemon juice over the dolmades. Cook for 10 minutes. Remove from the heat, cover, and let rest for 15 minutes.

7. The dolmades can be eaten warm, room temperature, or cold. Refrigerate any leftovers in an airtight container in the refrigerator for up to 5 days.

Per serving: 87 calories, 1 g protein, 8 g carbohydrates, 1 g sugars, 6 g total fat, 1 g saturated fat, 2 g fiber, 399 mg sodium

HUMMUS

Hummus is the blank slate of the dip world. It's terrific on its own with veggies or Whole Wheat Pitas (page 164), but it's also terrifically versatile (see variations below).

PREP TIME: 5 MINUTES / TOTAL TIME: 10 MINUTES / SERVES 8

1   can (15 ounces) chickpeas, drained and rinsed, or 1½ cups cooked and cooled chickpeas (see note on page 80)
¼   cup tahini
2   tablespoons extra-virgin olive oil
2   tablespoons fresh lemon juice
1   clove garlic, chopped
½   teaspoon ground cumin
½   teaspoon kosher salt

In a food processor or blender, combine the chickpeas, tahini, oil, lemon juice, garlic, cumin, and salt. Process until smooth, adding water, 1 tablespoon at a time, if necessary, to achieve desired consistency. Store in an airtight container in the refrigerator for up to 1 week.

Per serving: 106 calories, 3 g protein, 7 g carbohydrates, 0 g sugars, 8 g total fat, 1 g saturated fat, 2 g fiber, 244 mg sodium

149

VARIATIONS: Try changing out the chickpeas with any variety of your favorite bean (navy beans, cranberry beans, fava beans). Sprinkle a different topping on the finished hummus (black olives, pine nuts, feta cheese, olive oil drizzle). Or add any of the following to the food processor while blending the hummus.

¼ cup fresh herbs, such as parsley and/or mint
½ pound carrots, steamed or roasted until tender
½ cup oil-packed sundried tomatoes
1½ cups baby spinach
2 cups purple cauliflower florets, steamed

1 avocado
½ pound beets, steamed or roasted until tender
1 roasted red pepper
½ cup quartered water-packed artichoke hearts

CHICKPEAS

Pass the hummus, please! Meals based on vegetable protein sources such as chickpeas are actually more satiating than meals where the primary protein is meat, according to a recent Dutch study.[1] Since they're loaded with protein and fiber, chickpeas—as with other legumes and beans—fill you right up. That's a big reason why adding ¾ cup of beans to your diet every day could help you lose up to half a pound in just 6 weeks without making any other changes, found an *American Journal of Clinical Nutrition* analysis of more than 20 studies.[2] To top it all off, findings suggest that picking beans over burgers (or other types of red meat) most of the time could lower your cholesterol, slash your risk for heart disease, and even help you live longer.[3]

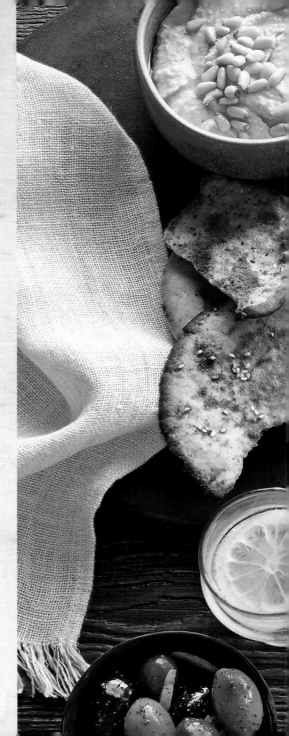

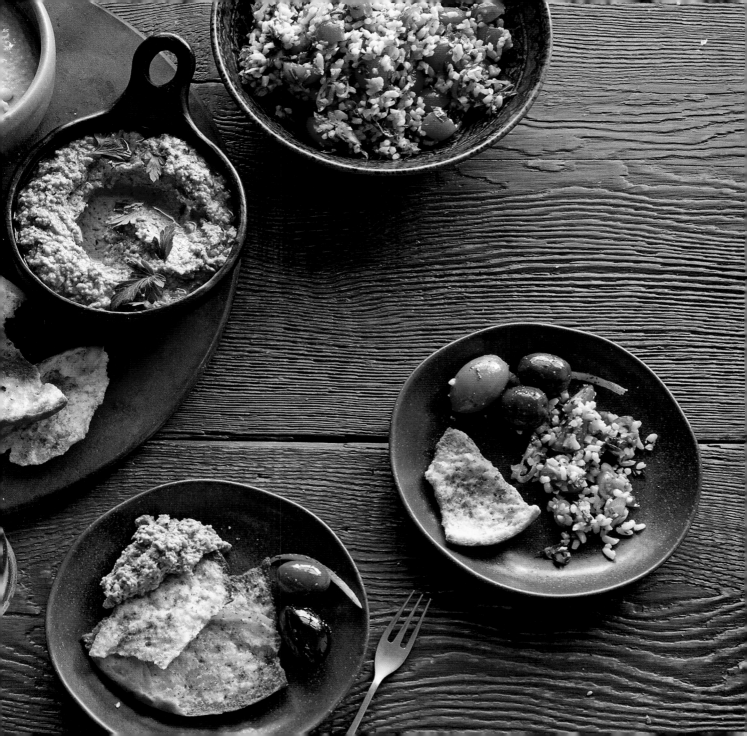

CRISPY SPICED CHICKPEAS

These crunchy, flavorful chickpeas are a healthier alternative to salty packaged snacks like chips or crackers. Have them as a snack, or serve them as a premeal nibble like you would olives or nuts.

PREP TIME: 5 MINUTES / TOTAL TIME: 30 MINUTES / SERVES 6

3   cans (15 ounces each) chickpeas, drained and rinsed (see note on page 80)
1   cup olive oil
1   teaspoon paprika
½   teaspoon ground cumin
½   teaspoon kosher salt
¼   teaspoon ground cinnamon
¼   teaspoon ground black pepper

1. Spread the chickpeas on paper towels and pat dry.

2. In a large saucepan over medium-high heat, warm the oil until shimmering. Add 1 chickpea; if it sizzles right away, the oil is hot enough to proceed.

3. Add enough chickpeas to form a single layer in the saucepan. Cook, occasionally gently shaking the saucepan until golden brown, about 8 minutes. With a slotted spoon, transfer to a paper towel–lined plate to drain. Repeat with the remaining chickpeas until all the chickpeas are fried. Transfer to a large bowl.

4. In a small bowl, combine the paprika, cumin, salt, cinnamon, and pepper. Sprinkle all over the fried chickpeas and toss to coat. The chickpeas will crisp as they cool.

Per serving: 175 calories, 6 g protein, 20 g carbohydrates, 2 g sugars, 9 g total fat, 1 g saturated fat, 5 g fiber, 509 mg sodium

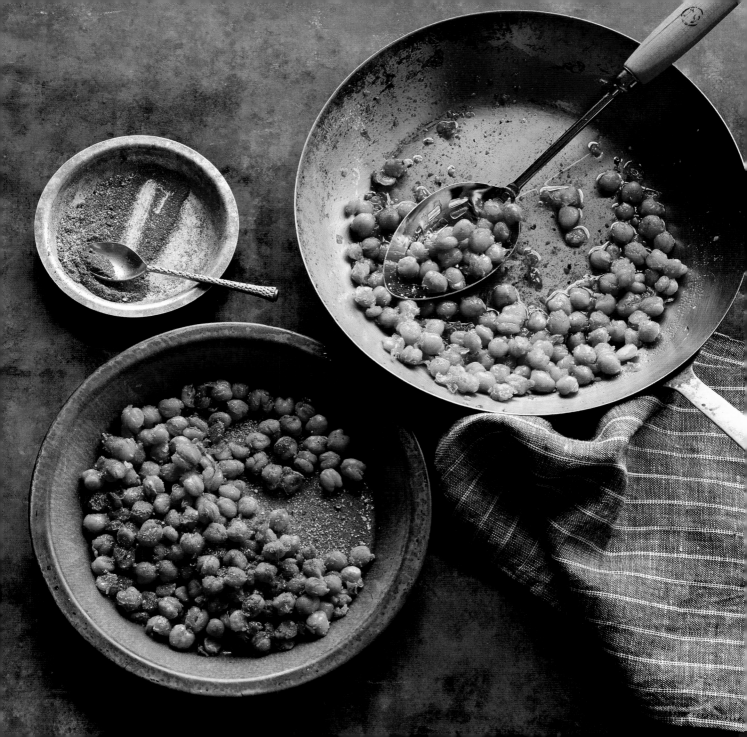

BABA GHANOUSH

This ubiquitous dip is a good way to convert eggplant haters to eggplant lovers. The smoky, garlicky spread is great as part of a meze plate (see page 123), spread in a sandwich, or served with crudités.

PREP TIME: 5 MINUTES / TOTAL TIME: 45 MINUTES / SERVES 6

1   eggplant, halved lengthwise
¼   cup tahini
2   tablespoons fresh lemon juice
1   clove garlic, chopped
¼   teaspoon kosher salt, plus more to taste
¼   teaspoon ground black pepper, plus more to taste
Extra-virgin olive oil, for serving (optional)
Chopped fresh flat-leaf parsley or cilantro,
    for serving (optional)

1. Preheat the oven to 400°F. Grease a baking sheet with olive oil.

2. Place the eggplant cut side down on the baking sheet. Roast until the skin is wrinkly and it has slightly collapsed, about 40 minutes. Remove from the oven and let cool until easily handled. Scoop the flesh from the eggplant and discard the skins.

3. In a food processor, add the eggplant, tahini, lemon juice, garlic, salt, and pepper and process until smooth and creamy. You may need to add 1 to 2 teaspoons of olive oil to get a smooth dip. Season to taste with the salt and pepper. To serve, spread the dip in a wide, shallow bowl. Drizzle with the oil and sprinkle with the herbs, if using.

Per serving: 80 calories, 3 g protein, 7 g carbohydrates, 3 g sugars, 5 g total fat, 1 g saturated fat, 3 g fiber, 102 mg sodium

154

BRAVAS-STYLE POTATOES

This classic Spanish dish is perfect for tapas-style entertaining. *Bravas* means "angry," and these potatoes get their fiery kick from red-pepper flakes and hot paprika. If the heat's too much, swap the hot paprika with smoked and omit the red-pepper flakes. Traditionally made with potatoes that are fried until crisp, we've baked ours to keep the fat in check.

PREP TIME: 15 MINUTES / TOTAL TIME: 1 HOUR 10 MINUTES / SERVES 8

- 4 large russet potatoes (about 2½ pounds), scrubbed and cut into 1" cubes
- 4 teaspoons olive oil, divided
- 1 teaspoon kosher salt, divided
- ½ teaspoon ground black pepper
- ¼ teaspoon red-pepper flakes
- ½ small yellow onion, chopped
- 1 large tomato, chopped
- 1 tablespoon sherry vinegar
- 1 teaspoon hot paprika
- 1 tablespoon chopped fresh flat-leaf parsley
  Hot sauce (optional)

1. Preheat the oven to 450°F. Bring a large pot of well-salted water to a boil.

2. Boil the potatoes until just barely tender, 5 to 8 minutes. Drain and transfer the potatoes to a large rimmed baking sheet. Add 1 tablespoon of the oil, ½ teaspoon of the salt, the black pepper, and pepper flakes. With 2 large spoons, toss very well to coat the potatoes in the oil. Spread the potatoes out on the baking sheet. Roast until the bottoms are starting to brown and crisp, 20 minutes. Carefully flip the potatoes and roast until the other side is golden and crisp, 15 to 20 minutes.

3. Meanwhile, in a small skillet over medium heat, warm the remaining 1 teaspoon oil. Cook the onion until softened, 3 to 4 minutes. Add the tomato and cook until it's broken down and saucy, 5 minutes. Stir in the vinegar, paprika, and the remaining ½ teaspoon salt. Cook for 30 seconds, remove from the heat, and cover to keep warm.

4. Transfer the potatoes to a large serving bowl. Drizzle the tomato mixture over the potatoes. Sprinkle with the parsley. Serve with hot sauce, if using.

Per serving: 173 calories, 4 g protein, 35 g carbohydrates, 2 g sugars, 2 g total fat, 0.5 g saturated fat, 3 g fiber, 251 mg sodium

HERB & SPICE DIPPING OILS

Flavored oils are an elegant and easy way to enjoy the benefits of olive oil. Most flavored oils shouldn't be stored because they will not keep well, so make small batches and use them immediately.

PREP TIME: 5 MINUTES / TOTAL TIME: 5 MINUTES / SERVES 6 TO 8

Herbs and spices (see below)
½ cup extra-virgin olive oil
Whole Wheat Pitas (page 164) or
    whole grain baguette, for serving
Flaky sea salt, such as Maldon, for serving
Ground black pepper, for serving

Serve the dipping oils with pita wedges or baguette slices, flaky sea salt, and ground black pepper.

VARIATIONS:

ROSEMARY GARLIC: Stir 1 tablespoon chopped fresh rosemary and 1 chopped clove garlic into the oil.

Per serving: 169 calories, 0 g protein, 0 g carbohydrates, 0 g sugars, 19 g total fat, 3 g saturated fat, 0 g fiber, 0 g sodium

THYME CORIANDER: Stir 1 tablespoon chopped fresh thyme and ½ teaspoon ground coriander into the oil.

Per serving: 169 calories, 0 g protein, 0 g carbohydrates, 0 g sugars, 19 g total fat, 3 g saturated fat, 0 g fiber, 0 g sodium

PARSLEY TOMATO: Stir 1 tablespoon chopped fresh flat-leaf parsley and 1 tablespoon chopped sun-dried tomatoes into the oil.

Per serving: 170 calories, 0 g protein, 0 g carbohydrates, 0 g sugars, 19 g total fat, 3 g saturated fat, 0 g fiber, 0 g sodium

OREGANO PEPPER: Stir 1 tablespoon chopped fresh oregano and ½ teaspoon ground black pepper into the oil.

Per serving: 169 calories, 0 g protein, 0 g carbohydrates, 0 g sugars, 19 g total fat, 3 g saturated fat, 0 g fiber, 0 g sodium

DILL SUMAC: Stir 1 tablespoon chopped fresh dill and ½ teaspoon ground sumac into the oil.

Per serving: 169 calories, 0 g protein, 0 g carbohydrates, 0 g sugars, 19 g total fat, 3 g saturated fat, 0 g fiber, 0 g sodium

MINT ZA'ATAR: Stir 1 tablespoon chopped fresh mint and 1 teaspoon za'atar into the oil.

Per serving: 169 calories, 0 g protein, 0 g carbohydrates, 0 g sugars, 19 g total fat, 3 g saturated fat, 0 g fiber, 0 g sodium

GRILLED NORTH AFRICAN SPICE-KISSED SWEET POTATOES

Warming spices like cinnamon, cumin, and coriander add a hint of sweet, smoky depth to this satisfying dish. Serve sweet potatoes as a side to roast chicken, or pair them with Greek yogurt for breakfast or a snack.

PREP TIME: 5 MINUTES / TOTAL TIME: 25 MINUTES / SERVES 8

¼   cup olive oil
3   cloves garlic, mashed to a paste
I   teaspoon kosher salt
I   teaspoon ground cumin
½   teaspoon ground coriander
¼   teaspoon ground cinnamon
    Pinch of cayenne pepper
2   pounds sweet potatoes, scrubbed and cut
    into ½"-thick wedges
¼   cup finely chopped fresh flat-leaf parsley
¼   cup pitted kalamata olives, slivered

1. Coat a grill rack or grill pan with olive oil and prepare the grill to medium-high heat.

2. In a large bowl, combine the oil, garlic, salt, cumin, coriander, cinnamon, and pepper. Toss in the sweet potato wedges until completely coated.

3. Grill the sweet potatoes until pronounced grill marks form on all sides and the wedges are completely tender, 3 to 6 minutes per side.

4. Transfer to a serving platter. Pour any remaining oil from the bowl over the potatoes and top with the parsley and olives.

Per serving: 179 calories, 2 g protein, 22 g carbohydrates, 6 g sugars, 10 g total fat, 1 g saturated fat, 4 g fiber, 466 mg sodium

157

NOTE: Bring these potatoes inside to the broiler and cook them the same way.

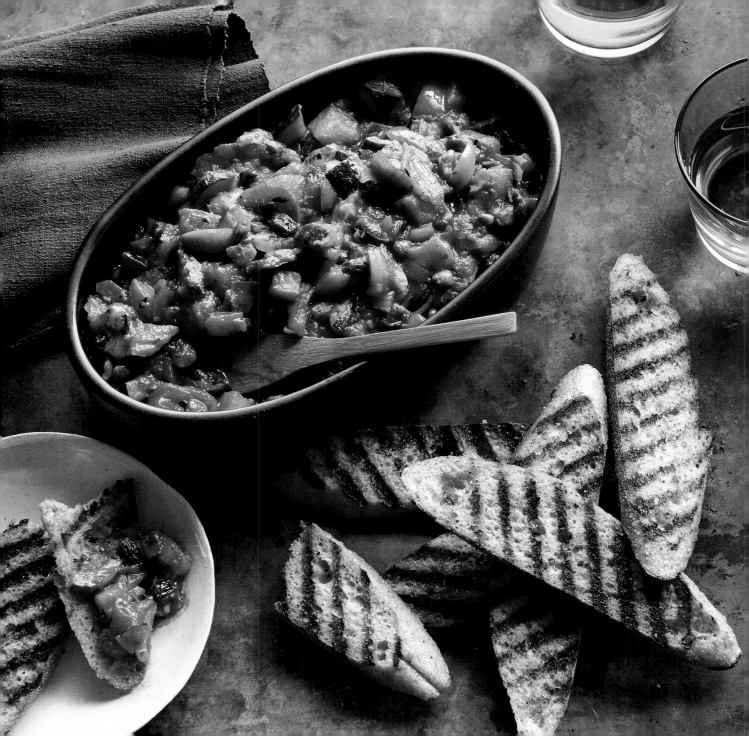

MIXED-VEGETABLE CAPONATA

Eggplant, zucchini, bell peppers, and onions turn rich, soft, and silky after slow-roasting in the oven. Serve this sweet summer veggie dish on whole grain toasts with scrambled eggs, or even stirred into yogurt.

PREP TIME: 15 MINUTES / TOTAL TIME: 55 MINUTES PLUS COOLING TIME / SERVES 8

1 eggplant, chopped
1 zucchini, chopped
1 red bell pepper, seeded and chopped
1 small red onion, chopped
2 tablespoons extra-virgin olive oil, divided
1 cup canned tomato sauce
3 tablespoons red wine vinegar
1 tablespoon honey
¼ teaspoon red-pepper flakes
¼ teaspoon kosher salt
½ cup pitted, chopped green olives
2 tablespoons drained capers
2 tablespoons raisins
2 tablespoons chopped fresh flat-leaf parsley

1. Preheat the oven to 400°F.

2. On a large rimmed baking sheet, toss the eggplant, zucchini, bell pepper, and onion with 1 tablespoon of the oil. Roast until the vegetables are tender, about 30 minutes.

3. In a medium saucepan over medium heat, warm the remaining 1 tablespoon oil. Add the tomato sauce, vinegar, honey, pepper flakes, and salt and stir to combine. Add the roasted vegetables, olives, capers, raisins, and parsley and cook until bubbly and thickened, 10 minutes.

4. Remove from the heat and cool to room temperature. Serve immediately or store in an airtight container in the refrigerator for up to 1 week.

Per serving: 100 calories, 2 g protein, 13 g carbohydrates,
8 g sugars, 5 g total fat, 1 g saturated fat, 4 g fiber,
464 mg sodium

159

FRIED BABY ARTICHOKES WITH LEMON-GARLIC AIOLI

Baby artichokes are sweeter and more tender than their larger cousins. They're easier to prep, too, since you don't have to remove the tough inner choke.

PREP TIME: 5 MINUTES / TOTAL TIME: I HOUR I5 MINUTES / SERVES I0

ARTICHOKES

I5 baby artichokes
½ lemon
3 cups olive oil
   Kosher salt, to taste

AIOLI

I egg
2 cloves garlic, chopped
I tablespoon fresh lemon juice
½ teaspoon Dijon mustard
½ cup olive oil
   Kosher salt and ground black pepper, to taste

1. *To make the artichokes:* Wash and drain the artichokes. With a paring knife, strip off the coarse outer leaves around the base and stalk, leaving the softer leaves on. Carefully peel the stalks and trim off all but 2" below the base. Slice off the top ½" of the artichokes. Cut each artichoke in half. Rub the cut surfaces with a lemon half to keep from browning.

2. In a medium saucepan fitted with a deep-fry thermometer over medium heat, warm the oil to about 280°F. Working in batches, cook the artichokes in the hot oil until tender, about 15 minutes. Using a slotted spoon, remove and drain on a paper towel–lined plate. Repeat with all the artichoke halves.

(continued)

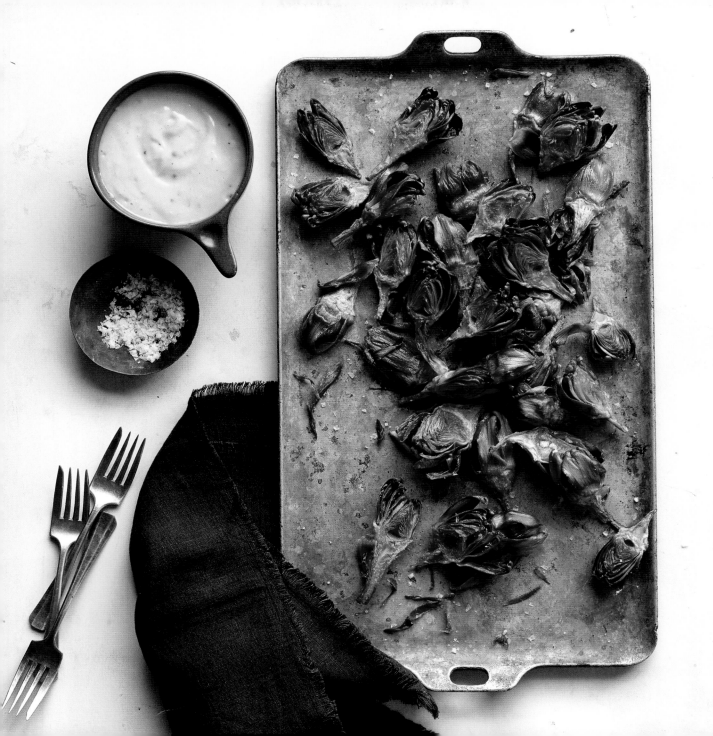

(continued from page 160)

3. Increase the heat of the oil to 375°F. In batches, cook the precooked baby artichokes until browned at the edges and crisp, about 1 minute. Transfer to a paper towel–lined plate. Season with the salt to taste. Repeat with the remaining artichokes.

4. ***To make the aioli:*** In a blender, pulse together the egg, garlic, lemon juice, and mustard until combined. With the blender running, slowly drizzle in the oil a few drops at a time until the mixture thickens like mayonnaise, about 2 minutes. Transfer to a bowl and season to taste with the salt and pepper.

5. Serve the warm artichokes with the aioli on the side.

Per serving: 236 calories, 6 g protein, 21 g carbohydrates, 2 g sugars, 17 g total fat, 3 g saturated fat, 10 g fiber, 283 mg sodium

MIXED-OLIVE TAPENADE

As delicious as this tapenade is, note that a serving is just 2 tablespoons. Spread it on crostini, crackers, or Whole Wheat Pitas (page 164) with a spot of goat cheese, if desired, or turn it into a quick lunch with a serving of pasta. While anchovies might not suit every palate, their presence brings a briny meatiness to this Provençal treat; feel free to omit them, though.

PREP TIME: 5 MINUTES / TOTAL TIME: 10 MINUTES / SERVES 8

1   cup (about 6 ounces) pitted black olives (such as kalamata and Niçoise)
1   cup (about 6 ounces) pitted green olives (such as Castelvetrano or Picholine)
1   tablespoon drained capers
1   anchovy fillet
    Juice of ½ lemon
1   tablespoon coarsely chopped fresh basil
2   teaspoons fresh thyme leaves
½   teaspoon dried marjoram or rosemary
1   clove garlic, chopped
2   tablespoons extra-virgin olive oil

In a food processor, combine the olives, capers, anchovy, lemon juice, basil, thyme, marjoram or rosemary, and garlic. Process or pulse as desired—less to keep it chunky, more to make it pasty and spreadable. Pulse in the olive oil until combined. Transfer to an airtight container and store in the refrigerator for up to 1 week.

Per serving: 172 calories, 1 g protein, 6 g carbohydrates, 0 g sugars, 17 g total fat, 2 g saturated fat, 0 g fiber, 1,000 mg sodium

163

NOTE: To add a pop of color, experiment with adding 3 or 4 chopped sun-dried tomatoes or ½ roasted red pepper into the food processor with the bulk of the ingredients.

WHOLE WHEAT PITAS

This traditional Mediterranean staple is the perfect bread for sandwiches, like Baked Falafel with Tzatziki Sauce, page 134; or salads, like Fattoush (*Lebanese Pita Salad*), page 119; or snacking with Hummus, page 149, or Mixed-Olive Tapenade, page 163.

PREP TIME: 5 MINUTES / TOTAL TIME: 2 HOURS 10 MINUTES / MAKES 8

2   cups whole wheat flour
1¼ cups all-purpose flour
1¼ teaspoons table salt
1¼ cup warm water (105°–110°F)
1   package (¼ ounce) active dry yeast (2½ teaspoons)
1   teaspoon olive oil

1. In the bowl of an electric stand mixer (or a large bowl), whisk together the flours and salt. In a small bowl or glass measuring cup, whisk together the water and yeast until the yeast is dissolved. Let sit until foamy, about 5 minutes. Add the yeast mixture to the flour mixture. Fit the mixer with the dough hook and mix on low (or stir) until it forms a shaggy dough.

2. Increase the speed to medium and knead until the dough is smooth and elastic, 2 to 3 minutes. If kneading by hand, turn the dough out onto a lightly floured work surface and knead about 10 minutes.

3. Form the dough into a ball and return it to the bowl. Pour in the oil, turning the dough to coat. Cover the bowl with a kitchen towel and let the dough rise until doubled in size, about 1 hour.

4. Preheat the oven to 475°F. Place a baking sheet on the lowest rack of the oven.

5. When the dough has risen, take it out of the bowl and give it a few gentle kneads. Divide the dough into 8 equal portions and shape into balls. Place on a lightly floured surface and cover with the kitchen towel.

6. Roll out each dough ball to form a 6" circle. Place on the heated baking sheet. Bake until puffed up and beginning to turn color, 6 to 7 minutes. Remove with a metal spatula or tongs and place in a bread basket or on a serving platter. Repeat with the remaining dough balls.

7. To make a pocket in the pita, allow it to cool. Slice off $\frac{1}{4}$ of the pita from 1 edge, and then carefully insert the knife into the pita to cut the pocket. Gently pull the sides apart to make the pocket larger.

Per serving: 181 calories, 6 g protein, 37 g carbohydrates, 0 g sugars, 2 g total fat, 0 g saturated fat, 4 g fiber, 366 mg sodium

NOTE: Pitas freeze well, but they also make great pita chips, strips, and croutons. Cut each pita into eighths or strips, drizzle with olive oil, and sprinkle with za'atar spice or grated Parmigiano-Reggiano cheese. Place on a baking sheet and toast in a 400°F oven until golden, about 5 minutes.

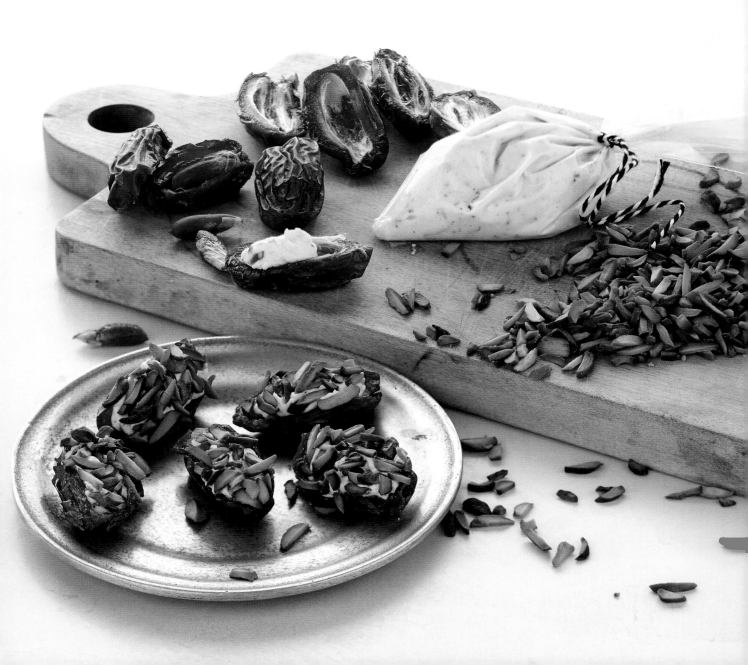

CHEESE-STUFFED DATES

If you can't find dates, try Calimyrna figs instead. If your fruit is very dry and hard to work with, rehydrate it by soaking it in hot water for 5 minutes. Drain and pat dry before proceeding.

PREP TIME: 10 MINUTES / TOTAL TIME: 20 MINUTES / SERVES 4

2   ounces low-fat cream cheese, at room temperature
2   tablespoons sweet pickle relish
1   tablespoon low-fat plain Greek yogurt
1   teaspoon finely chopped fresh chives
¼   teaspoon kosher salt
⅛   teaspoon ground black pepper
    Dash of hot sauce
2   tablespoons pistachios, chopped
8   medjool dates, pitted and halved

1. In a small bowl, stir together the cream cheese, relish, yogurt, chives, salt, pepper, and hot sauce.

2. Put the pistachios on a clean plate. Put the cream cheese mixture into a resealable plastic bag, and snip off 1 corner of the bag. Pipe the cream cheese mixture into the date halves and press the tops into the pistachios to coat.

Per serving: 196 calories, 3 g protein, 41 g carbohydrates, 35 g sugars, 4 g total fat, 1.5 g saturated fat, 4 g fiber, 294 mg sodium

167

ROSEMARY-GRAPE FOCACCIA

Focaccia is an Italian flatbread made from a yeasted dough that takes extra time for I additional rise, or proof. Here, we simplify this classic with store-bought pizza dough. Choose dough that comes in bags, rather than peel-and-pop canisters.

PREP TIME: 5 MINUTES / TOTAL TIME: 50 MINUTES / SERVES 8

I   pound whole wheat pizza dough
3   tablespoons olive oil or grape-seed oil, divided
I   tablespoon fresh rosemary, chopped
½   teaspoon kosher salt
I   cup red or black seedless grapes, halved
2   tablespoons pine nuts
    Generous pinch of flaky sea salt, such as Maldon (optional)

1. Preheat the oven to 400°F. Set out the dough at room temperature for 10 minutes.

2. Meanwhile, in a small saucepan over medium-low heat, combine 2 tablespoons of the oil, the rosemary, and kosher salt and warm for 5 minutes. Remove from the heat and set aside to steep.

3. Brush a rimmed baking sheet with the remaining 1 tablespoon oil. Press the dough into the baking sheet, stretching it out 10" to 12" in diameter. With your fingers, make dimples in the dough, and brush it with some of the rosemary oil. Sprinkle the grapes and pine nuts over the dough, pushing the grapes in a little bit. Generously brush the top with the remaining rosemary oil. Sprinkle with the flaky sea salt, if using.

4. Bake until the dough is golden, 20 to 25 minutes. Cool 10 minutes before cutting and serving.

Per serving: 192 calories, 4 g protein, 28 g carbohydrates, 3 g sugars, 9 g total fat, 1 g saturated fat, 4 g fiber, 369 mg sodium

GRAPES

Just like red wine, these juicy fruits are a top source of resveratrol—the antioxidant compound thought to support heart health by lowering bad cholesterol, promoting healthy blood pressure, and reducing the risk for blood clots and blood vessel damage.[4] Grapes are also rich in anthocyanins, another family of heart-healthy polyphenols. And, according to one Harvard study, eating 3 servings of anthocyanin-rich fruits per week could reduce heart attack risk by as much as 34 percent.[5] Choose red, purple, or black grapes for the biggest benefit—they pack more antioxidant power than their green counterparts.

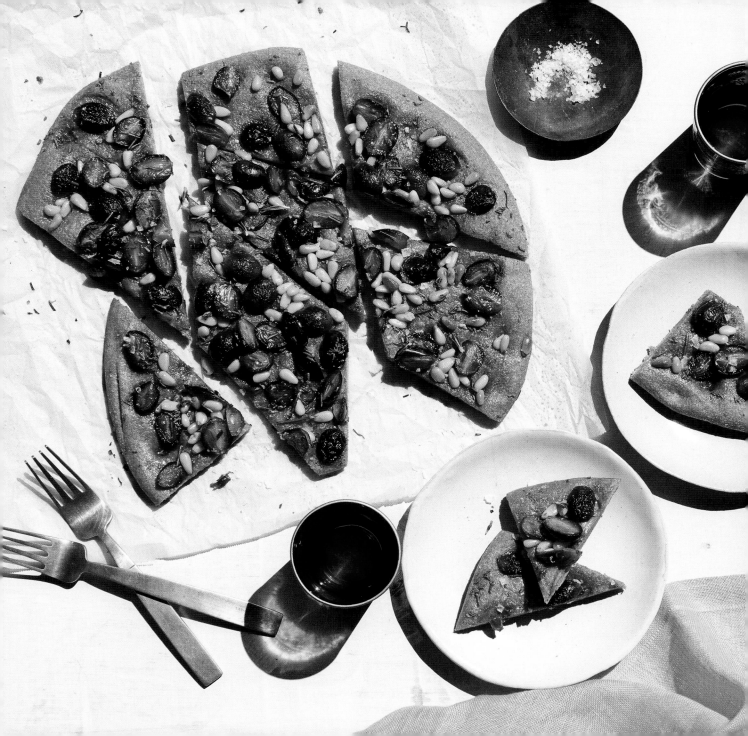

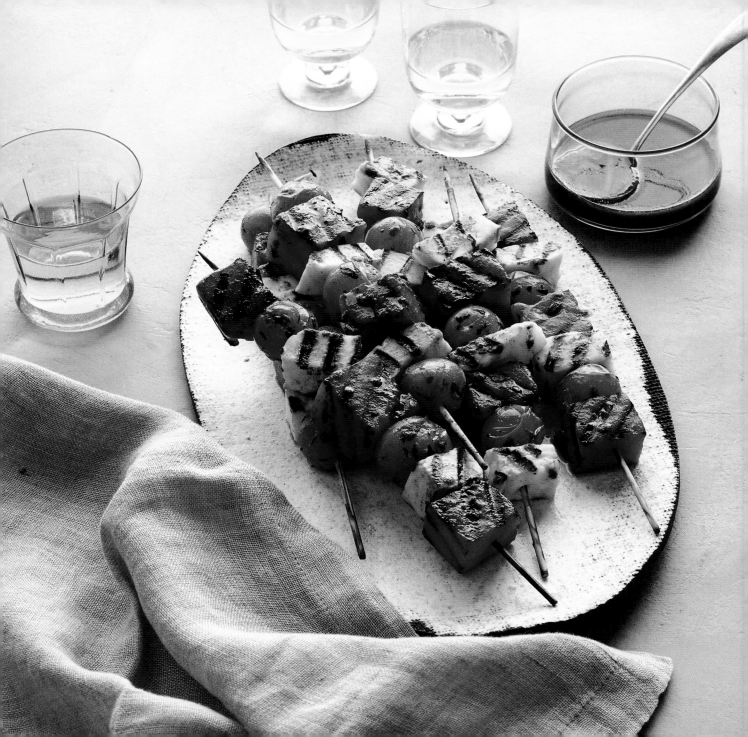

HALLOUMI, WATERMELON, TOMATO KEBABS WITH BASIL OIL DRIZZLE

Halloumi is a firm, salty cheese from Cyprus made from sheep's and goat's milk. It is lower in fat than many cheeses and won't melt on the grill. Look for it in well-stocked grocery stores or specialty cheese shops.

PREP TIME: 20 MINUTES / TOTAL TIME: 30 MINUTES / SERVES 8

¼ cup coarsely chopped fresh basil
3 tablespoons extra-virgin olive oil
I small clove garlic, chopped
¼ teaspoon kosher salt
¼ teaspoon ground black pepper
32 cubes (I½") watermelon (from I melon)
32 cherry tomatoes (about I½ pints)
I package (8–10 ounces) Halloumi cheese, cut into 32 cubes (¾"–I")

1. Soak 16 skewers (6" or 8") in water.
2. In a blender or food processor, combine the basil, oil, garlic, salt, and pepper. Blend until the basil is finely chopped and the mixture is well combined.
3. Alternately thread the watermelon, tomatoes, and cheese onto the skewers. Brush with half the basil oil. Coat a grill rack or grill pan with olive oil and prepare the grill to medium-high heat.
4. Grill the kebabs, covered, until good grill marks form on the cheese, about 8 minutes, turning once.
5. Set kebabs on a platter and drizzle with the remaining basil oil.

Per serving: 178 calories, 7 g protein, 6 g carbohydrates, 5 g sugars, 15 g total fat, 6 g saturated fat, 1 g fiber, 365 mg sodium

171

NOTE: If you have a pot of mint growing in your yard, feel free to swap it for the basil in the drizzling oil. Combining the basil and mint would also be delicious.

BASIC PESTO

This recipe is a great way to preserve your summer basil, and it freezes well. Portion in an ice cube tray, freeze, and then transfer to a resealable plastic freezer bag. Defrost what you need in the refrigerator overnight.

PREP TIME: 5 MINUTES / TOTAL TIME: 10 MINUTES / SERVES 6

4 cups basil leaves
¼ cup pine nuts
1 clove garlic, minced
¼ teaspoon kosher salt
¼ cup extra-virgin olive oil
¼ cup shredded Parmigiano-Reggiano cheese

In a food processor, add the basil, pine nuts, garlic, and salt and pulse a few times to break down into coarse pieces. With the food processor running, stream in the oil. Scrape down the sides of the bowl and pulse once more. Stir in the cheese. Use immediately, or store in an airtight container with plastic wrap pressed directly on the surface in the refrigerator for up to 1 week. Bring the pesto to room temperature before using on pasta or for other recipes.

Per serving: 135 calories, 2 g protein, 1 g carbohydrates, 0 g sugars, 14 g total fat, 2.5 g saturated fat, 0 g fiber, 117 mg sodium

172

VARIATIONS: Mix and match ingredients to create your own custom nontraditional "pesto" flavor combinations.

✣ Replace the basil with flat-leaf parsley, kale, mint, arugula, cilantro, or peeled broccoli stems.

✣ Replace the pine nuts with pistachios, macadamia nuts, pecans, walnuts, almonds, or cashews.

✣ Possible combos: parsley and walnut, kale and cashew, mint and pistachio, arugula and almond, cilantro and macadamia, broccoli stems and pecan.

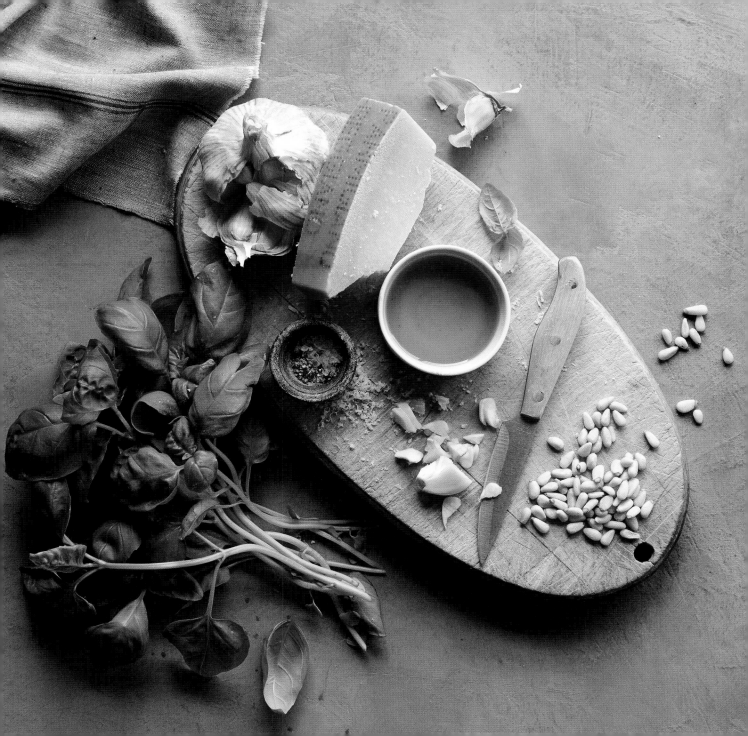

ONE-PAN HERB-ROASTED TOMATOES, GREEN BEANS, AND BABY POTATOES

This side is a simple way to get a few veggies and a starch on the table in one fell swoop. It's easy enough for weeknight dinners—but elegant enough for parties and gatherings.

PREP TIME: 10 MINUTES / TOTAL TIME: 40 MINUTES / SERVES 6

¼ cup chopped mixed fresh herbs, such as flat-leaf parsley, oregano, mint, and dill
3 tablespoons olive oil
½ teaspoon kosher salt
½ teaspoon ground black pepper
1 pound baby potatoes, halved
1 pound green beans, trimmed and halved
2 large shallots, cut into wedges
2 pints cherry tomatoes

1. Preheat the oven to 400°F.
2. In a small bowl, whisk together the herbs, oil, salt, and pepper. Place the potatoes, string beans, and shallots on a large rimmed baking sheet. Drizzle the herb mixture over the vegetables and toss thoroughly to coat.
3. Roast the vegetables until the potatoes are just tender, about 15 minutes. Remove from the oven and toss in the tomatoes. Roast until the tomatoes blister and the potatoes are completely tender, about 15 minutes.

Per serving: 173 calories, 5 g protein, 26 g carbohydrates, 7 g sugars, 8 g total fat, 1 g saturated fat, 5 g fiber, 185 mg sodium

CAULIFLOWER RICE PILAF

When processed to form tiny grainlike pieces, cauliflower makes a tasty stand-in for rice or other grains. Enjoy this as you would other pilafs—alongside fish or chicken or stuffed into vegetables.

PREP TIME: 10 MINUTES / TOTAL TIME: 35 MINUTES / SERVES 4

1 eggplant, diced
1½ tablespoons olive oil, divided
    Kosher salt and ground black pepper
1 large head cauliflower, trimmed
1 large shallot, finely chopped
¼ cup golden raisins
¼ cup pine nuts, toasted
¼ cup finely chopped fresh flat-leaf parsley
1 tablespoon grated lemon peel

1. Preheat the oven to 350°F.

2. On a large rimmed baking sheet, toss the eggplant with 1 tablespoon of the oil and season generously with the salt and pepper. Roast, tossing occasionally, until tender and golden, about 25 minutes.

3. Meanwhile, cut the cauliflower into 2" florets and transfer to a food processor. Pulse until the florets break down into even rice-size pieces.

4. In a large skillet over medium heat, warm the remaining ½ tablespoon oil until shimmering. Cook the shallot until translucent, about 5 minutes. Stir in the cauliflower rice and cook until tender, about 4 minutes.

5. Add the raisins, pine nuts, parsley, and lemon peel and stir to combine. Toss with the roasted eggplant and season to taste with the salt and pepper.

Per serving: 237 calories, 8 g protein, 31 g carbohydrates, 17 g sugars, 12 g total fat, 1 g saturated fat, 9 g fiber, 311 mg sodium

175

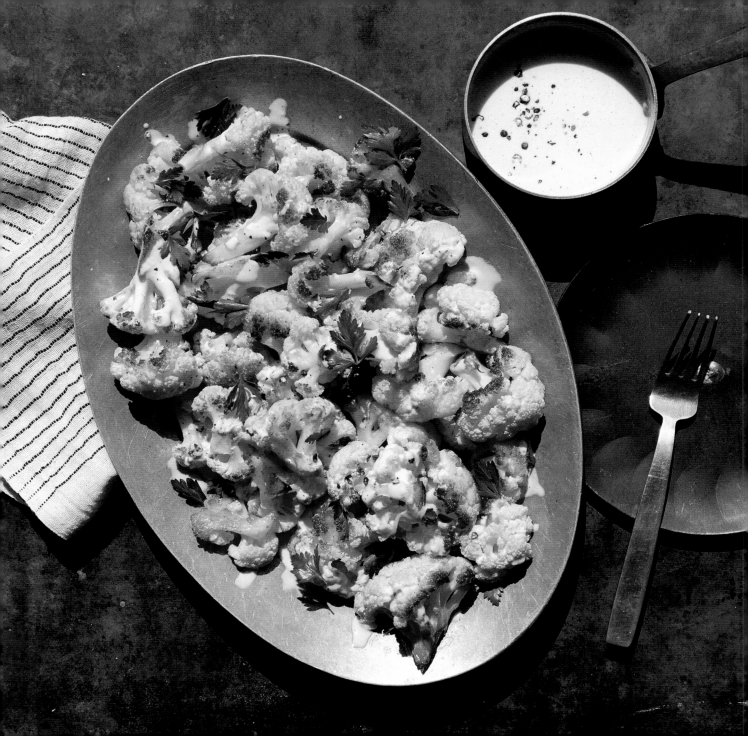

ARNABIT
(ROASTED CAULIFLOWER)
WITH SPICY TAHINI SAUCE

This dish, called arnabit in Arabic, is often fried. We've lightened it up by roasting the cauliflower to a golden brown deliciousness, which makes it perfectly suited for the tahini sauce with a garlicky kick.

PREP TIME: 10 MINUTES / TOTAL TIME: 45 MINUTES / SERVES 6

1   head cauliflower, cut into bite-size pieces
2   tablespoons olive oil
½   teaspoon kosher salt, divided
¼   cup tahini
3   tablespoons warm water
    Juice of 1 lemon
2   cloves garlic, minced
1   tablespoon chopped fresh flat-leaf parsley or mint

1. Preheat the oven to 425°F.

2. On a large rimmed baking sheet, toss the cauliflower with the oil. Season with half of the salt. Spread in an even layer and roast until deep golden brown, about 35 minutes.

3. Meanwhile, in a small bowl or food processor, combine the tahini, water, lemon juice, garlic, and the remaining salt. Stir or process until smooth, adding more water, 1 teaspoon at a time, if the mixture is too thick.

4. Transfer the cauliflower to a serving dish, drizzle with the tahini sauce, and sprinkle with the parsley or mint.

Per serving: 162 calories, 6 g protein, 15 g carbohydrates, 5 g sugars, 11 g total fat, 1.5 g saturated fat, 5 g fiber, 236 mg sodium

MUHAMMARA
(ROASTED RED PEPPER AND WALNUT DIP)

Muhammara is a roasted red pepper and walnut dip popular in Syria and Turkey, where it is prepared with hot peppers as well as bell peppers. Our version is decidedly mild, but you can increase the cayenne pepper if you'd like it spicier.

PREP TIME: 10 MINUTES / TOTAL TIME: 15 MINUTES / SERVES 6

1   jar (12 ounces) roasted red peppers, drained
1   cup walnuts, toasted
⅓   cup whole wheat bread crumbs
2   cloves garlic, chopped
2   tablespoons extra-virgin olive oil
2   teaspoons pomegranate molasses (see note on page 115)
1   teaspoon fresh lemon juice
1   teaspoon ground cumin
½   teaspoon kosher salt
¼   teaspoon ground black pepper
¼   teaspoon cayenne pepper (optional)
    Whole Wheat Pitas (page 164) or crudités, for serving

In a food processor, combine the roasted red peppers, walnuts, bread crumbs, garlic, oil, pomegranate molasses, lemon juice, cumin, salt, black pepper, and cayenne (if using). Pulse until a coarse puree forms. Serve with the pita or crudités.

Per serving: 258 calories, 5 g protein, 17 g carbohydrates, 2 g sugars, 18 g total fat, 2 g saturated fat, 2 g fiber, 706 mg sodium

STUFFED MINI PEPPERS

Filled with chicken, couscous, feta, and herbs, these flavorful peppers are practically a meal in themselves. But they're also a delicious addition to a snack or appetizer spread at parties.

PREP TIME: 10 MINUTES / TOTAL TIME: 50 MINUTES / SERVES 10 (3 PER SERVING)

15 multicolored mini bell peppers, halved and seeded
2 tablespoons olive oil, divided, plus more for drizzling
¾ cup whole wheat Israeli couscous
1 cup shredded rotisserie chicken, coarsely chopped
⅓ cup crumbled feta cheese
2 tablespoons lemon juice
2 tablespoons finely chopped fresh flat-leaf parsley
1 tablespoon finely chopped fresh oregano
1 tablespoon finely chopped fresh basil
1 clove garlic, mashed into a paste
   Kosher salt and ground black pepper, to taste

1. Preheat the oven to 400°F.

2. Place the pepper halves cut side up on a large rimmed baking sheet. Drizzle with 1 tablespoon of the oil and roast until tender but not soft, about 10 minutes. Remove from the oven and let cool to room temperature.

3. Cook the couscous according to package directions. Let cool slightly.

4. Stir the remaining 1 tablespoon oil, the chicken, cheese, lemon juice, herbs, and garlic into the couscous. Season to taste with the salt and black pepper.

5. Stuff each pepper with a rounded table-spoonful of the couscous mixture. Drizzle with a little olive oil.

Per serving: 136 calories, 6 g protein, 13 g carbohydrates, 2 g sugars, 7 g total fat, 2 g saturated fat, 2 g fiber, 173 mg sodium

SAFFRON COUSCOUS WITH ALMONDS, CURRANTS, AND SCALLIONS

Traditional Moroccan couscous is cooked in a tagine—a ceramic conelike pot that allows steam to rise, condense, and drip back down onto the food. We've simplified the process by steaming the couscous in a covered saucepan.

PREP TIME: 5 MINUTES / TOTAL TIME: 40 MINUTES / SERVES 8

2 cups whole wheat couscous
1 tablespoon olive oil
5 scallions, thinly sliced, whites and greens kept separate
1 large pinch saffron threads, crumbled
3 cups low-sodium chicken broth or vegetable broth
½ cup slivered almonds
¼ cup dried currants
Kosher salt and ground black pepper, to taste

1. In a medium saucepan over medium heat, toast the couscous, stirring occasionally, until lightly browned, about 5 minutes. Transfer to a bowl.

2. In the same saucepan, add the oil and scallion whites. Cook, stirring, until lightly browned, about 5 minutes. Sprinkle in the saffron and stir to combine. Pour in the broth and bring to a boil.

3. Remove the saucepan from the heat, stir in the couscous, cover, and let sit until all the liquid is absorbed and the couscous is tender, about 15 minutes.

4. Fluff the couscous with a fork. Fluff in the scallion greens, almonds, and currants. Season to taste with the salt and pepper.

Per serving: 212 calories, 8 g protein, 34 g carbohydrates, 4 g sugars, 6 g total fat, 1 g saturated fat, 4 g fiber, 148 mg sodium

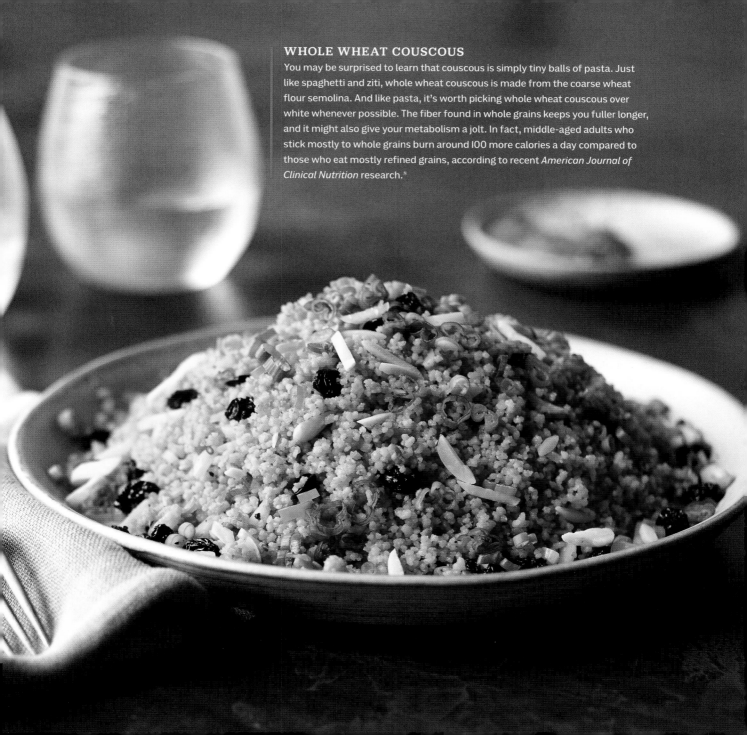

WHOLE WHEAT COUSCOUS

You may be surprised to learn that couscous is simply tiny balls of pasta. Just like spaghetti and ziti, whole wheat couscous is made from the coarse wheat flour semolina. And like pasta, it's worth picking whole wheat couscous over white whenever possible. The fiber found in whole grains keeps you fuller longer, and it might also give your metabolism a jolt. In fact, middle-aged adults who stick mostly to whole grains burn around 100 more calories a day compared to those who eat mostly refined grains, according to recent *American Journal of Clinical Nutrition* research.[8]

WARM BEETS WITH HAZELNUTS AND SPICED YOGURT

Cool, tangy yogurt is an ideal contrast for warm, earthy beets. Enjoy these as part of a meze plate (see page 123), or stuff them into a pita for a quick lunch.

PREP TIME: 5 MINUTES / TOTAL TIME: 45 MINUTES / SERVES 4

4   or 5 beets, peeled
¼   cup hazelnuts
½   cup low-fat plain Greek yogurt
1   tablespoon honey
1   tablespoon chopped fresh mint
1   teaspoon ground cinnamon
¼   teaspoon ground cumin
⅛   teaspoon ground black pepper

1. Place racks in the upper and lower thirds of the oven. Preheat the oven to 400°F.
2. Place the beets on a 12" x 12" piece of foil. Fold the foil over the beets, and seal the sides. Bake until the beets are tender enough to be pierced by a fork, about 40 minutes. Remove from the oven, carefully open the packet, and let cool slightly. When cool enough to handle, slice the beets into ¼"-thick rounds.

3. Meanwhile, toast the hazelnuts on a small baking sheet until browned and fragrant, about 5 minutes. Using a paper towel or kitchen towel, rub the skins off. Coarsely chop the nuts and set aside.
4. In a medium bowl, stir together the yogurt, honey, mint, cinnamon, cumin, and pepper.
5. Serve the beets with a dollop of the spiced yogurt and a sprinkle of the nuts.

Per serving: 126 calories, 5 g protein, 15 g carbohydrates, 11 g sugars, 6 g total fat, 1 g saturated fat, 4 g fiber, 74 mg sodium

YOGURT

Before the days of refrigeration, this fermented food may have merely been a convenient way to preserve milk longer. But now, we know that yogurt is also considerably more nutritious than its liquid counterpart. It packs more protein, vitamins, and minerals than milk, and the higher acidity levels can aid in the absorption of nutrients like calcium and magnesium. And because many of the milk sugars are already broken down, people with lactose intolerance are often able to enjoy it.

But the biggest draw might be yogurt's probiotics, or good bacteria. These friendly bugs are known to promote healthy digestion, but that's only the start. Probiotics are thought to guard the lining of the gut, helping to keep toxins and bacteria from entering the bloodstream and bolstering the immune system. That could offer more protection against everyday ailments like the cold or flu, as well as chronic conditions like eczema, allergies, and asthma. Probiotics are also thought to improve blood sugar regulation and fight inflammation, which could be why Harvard researchers discovered that a daily serving of yogurt—but not other forms of dairy—was linked to an 18 percent lower risk for type 2 diabetes.[7]

Which yogurt is best? Regular yogurt, thicker Greek yogurt, spreadable yogurt cheeses like labneh, tart Balkan sheep's milk yogurt, or even kefir are all good choices, so enjoy whatever you like best. Just be sure to stick with plain yogurt since flavored options tend to be high in added sugar, and look for products with "live active cultures" on the packaging. As for the fat content? Both full- and low-fat yogurt can be part of a healthy diet, so pick what works best for your nutritional goals. Low-fat yogurt might be a better option if you're trying to lose weight, simply because it's lower in calories.

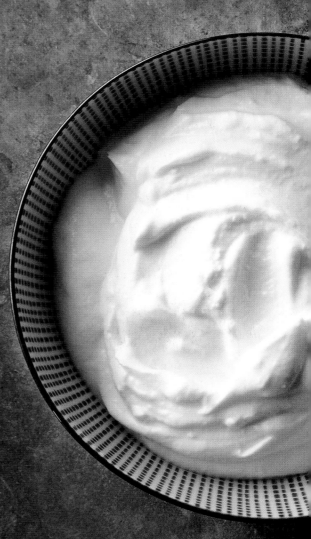

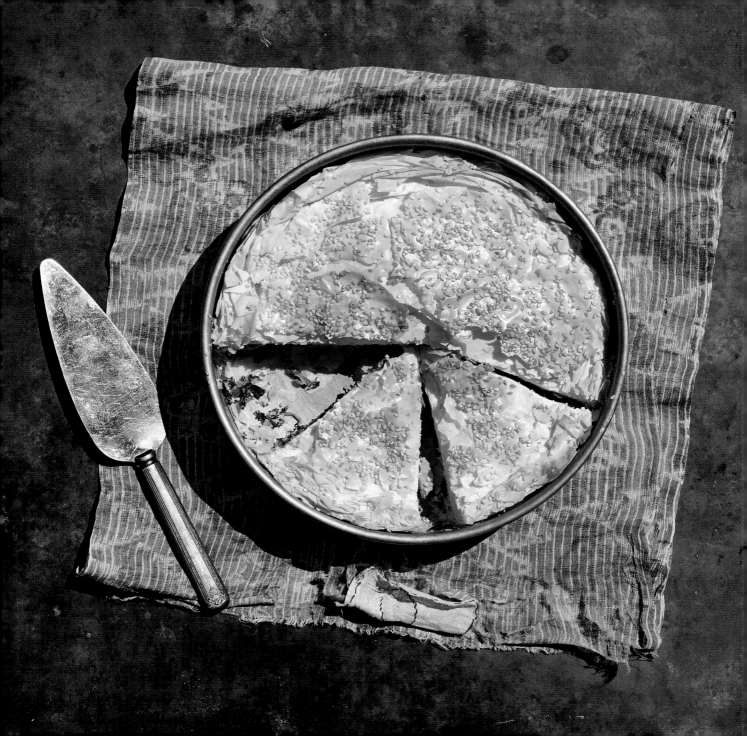

CRETAN GREENS PIE

If you can find any wild greens such as purslane, dandelion, or chickweed, use them in place of the chard. An easy alternative to brushing the olive oil over the phyllo dough is to use a nonaerosol olive oil spray.

PREP TIME: 10 MINUTES / TOTAL TIME: 1 HOUR 15 MINUTES / SERVES 6

2   teaspoons plus ¼ cup olive oil
6   scallions, thinly sliced
1   large leek, white and light green parts, sliced
7   cups (7 ounces) chopped fresh spinach
4   cups chopped chard (1 large bunch)
¼   cup chopped fresh chervil, flat-leaf parsley, or tarragon
1   egg
3   ounces feta cheese, crumbled
2   tablespoons chopped fresh dill
2   tablespoons chopped fresh mint
½   teaspoon kosher salt
¼   teaspoon ground black pepper
24   sheets phyllo dough, thawed if frozen
1   tablespoon sesame seeds

1. Place a rack in the lower third of the oven. Preheat the oven to 350°F.

2. In a medium skillet over medium heat, warm 2 teaspoons of the oil. Cook the scallions and leek until tender, about 5 minutes. Add the spinach, chard, and chervil, parsley, or tarragon and cook until wilted and bright green, about 3 minutes. Place the greens in a colander and let drain until cooled. When cooled, squeeze out and discard any remaining liquid and place the greens in a large bowl.

3. In a small bowl, beat the egg and stir in the cheese, dill, mint, salt, and pepper. Stir this mixture into the greens and mix well.

4. Lightly brush or spray the bottom of a 9" round cake pan with olive oil. Carefully separate 1 sheet of the phyllo and place it in the pan, allowing the phyllo to overlap the sides of the pan. Brush or spray with some of the ¼ cup oil and repeat for 11 more layers, rotating each layer to create an even crust up the sides of the pan.

5. Pour the greens mixture on top of the phyllo and spread out evenly. Fold the phyllo overhang in onto the filling.

6. Repeat the layering process with the remaining phyllo, tucking the edges in around the sides of the pan. Brush the top with some of the oil and sprinkle with the sesame seeds.

7. Bake until golden, 35 to 40 minutes. Serve warm or at room temperature.

Per serving: 404 calories, 10 g protein, 46 g carbohydrates, 2 g sugars, 20 g total fat, 5 g saturated fat, 3 g fiber, 807 mg sodium

185

TABBOULEH

No matter how you see it spelled, tabbouleh or tabouli is essentially an herb salad. It's typically made with lemon-dressed bulgur wheat—but think of the bulgur as the garnish, rather than as the main dish.

PREP TIME: 10 MINUTES / TOTAL TIME: 2 HOURS / SERVES 6

¾ cup bulgur wheat
¾ cup boiling-hot water
Juice of I lemon
3 tablespoons extra-virgin olive oil
I cup chopped fresh mint
I cup chopped fresh flat-leaf parsley
3 scallions, thinly sliced
½ pint cherry tomatoes or grape tomatoes, halved
I clove garlic, minced
½ teaspoon kosher salt
¼ teaspoon ground black pepper

1. In a large bowl, combine the bulgur and water. Cover and set aside until the liquid is absorbed and the bulgur is tender, 50 to 60 minutes.

2. Fluff the bulgur with a fork. Drizzle with the lemon juice and oil and toss again. Add the mint, parsley, and scallions and toss to thoroughly distribute. Add the tomatoes, garlic, salt, and pepper and toss again.

3. Set aside at room temperature for 1 hour to allow the flavors to blend, or refrigerate until ready to eat.

Per serving: 139 calories, 3 g protein, 17 g carbohydrates, 1 g sugars, 7 g total fat, 1 g saturated fat, 4 g fiber, 173 mg sodium

VARIATIONS: Play with this recipe and combine all of your favorite Mediterranean flavors into endless variations of the traditional version.

❋ Stuff the tabbouleh into 6 hollowed-out tomato or bell pepper halves. Bake, covered, at 375°F until the tomatoes or peppers are tender, 35 to 45 minutes.

❋ Omit the mint, parsley, and tomatoes. Add 2 cups shredded kale + 1 diced apple + $\frac{1}{4}$ cup chopped walnuts + $\frac{1}{4}$ cup pomegranate seeds.

❋ Add 1 chopped cucumber + $\frac{1}{4}$ cup chopped kalamata olives + 3 tablespoons crumbled feta cheese.

❋ Omit the bulgur and mint. Add 1 can (15 ounces) drained-and-rinsed chickpeas + 1 cup chopped fresh basil. Finish with 3 tablespoons freshly grated Parmigiano-Reggiano cheese.

❋ Replace the bulgur with $\frac{3}{4}$ cup dry quinoa, millet, or barley, cooked according to package directions.

❋ Omit the tomatoes and garlic. Add 1 cup pitted and halved cherries + $\frac{1}{4}$ cup chopped almonds.

❋ Omit the tomatoes. Add $\frac{1}{3}$ cup dried or 3 fresh apricots, chopped + $\frac{1}{4}$ cup chopped pistachios.

❋ Omit the tomatoes. Add 1 chopped peach + 2 ounces crumbed ricotta salata.

❋ Omit the lemon juice and salt. Add 1 chopped preserved lemon + $\frac{1}{4}$ cup raisins + 1 tablespoon za'atar spice.

❋ Omit the tomatoes, mint, and lemon juice. Add 1 cup chopped fresh cilantro + 1 chopped roasted red pepper + $\frac{1}{4}$ cup orange juice + $\frac{1}{4}$ cup chopped green olives.

BAKED TURKEY KIBBEH

Traditionally made with beef or lamb, we used turkey to help keep this recipe a touch more heart healthy but kept all the flavor. Make sure not to use 99% fat-free ground turkey because it will dry out—stick with ground turkey or ground turkey breast.

PREP TIME: 15 MINUTES / TOTAL TIME: OVERNIGHT SOAK PLUS 1 HOUR 20 MINUTES / SERVES 8

OUTER LAYER

- 1½ cups bulgur wheat
- 1¼ pounds ground turkey
- 1 yellow onion, grated on a box grater
- ½ cup finely chopped fresh mint
- 1 teaspoon ground allspice
- ½ teaspoon ground cinnamon
- 1 teaspoon kosher salt
- ¼ teaspoon ground black pepper

FILLING

- 4 tablespoons olive oil, divided
- 1 yellow onion, finely chopped
- 3 cloves garlic, minced
- 1 pound ground turkey
- ¼ cup finely chopped fresh flat-leaf parsley
- ½ cup pine nuts, toasted
- ½ teaspoon ground allspice
- ½ teaspoon kosher salt
- ¼ teaspoon ground black pepper

FOR ASSEMBLY AND SERVING

- 1 tablespoon olive oil
- 8 tablespoons low-fat Greek yogurt or labneh
- ¼ cup thinly sliced fresh mint

1. *To make the outer layer:* Soak the bulgur overnight in a bowl with enough water to cover by 2".

2. Drain, squeezing the bulgur until there is no excess moisture. Transfer to a large bowl.

3. With your hands, mix in the turkey, onion, mint, allspice, cinnamon, salt, and pepper until thoroughly combined.

4. *To make the filling:* In a medium cast-iron skillet over medium heat, warm 2 tablespoons of the oil. Cook the onion and garlic until translucent, about 8 minutes. Add the turkey and cook until no longer pink, about 5 minutes.

5. Stir in the parsley, pine nuts, allspice, salt, and pepper. Drizzle in the remaining 2 tablespoons oil. Transfer to a bowl and wipe out the skillet.

6. *To assemble the kibbeh:* Preheat an oven to 350°F. Lightly coat the cast-iron skillet with olive oil.

7. Press half of the outer layer into the bottom of the skillet in an even layer about ¾" thick. Spread the filling evenly over the top. Using wet fingers, use the remaining half of the outer layer to cover the filling. Once the filling is completely covered, smooth with wet hands.

8. Score the surface of the kibbeh into 8 wedges to make it easier to cut and portion after baking. Drizzle the oil over the top and bake until deep brown, about 30 minutes.

9. Serve hot with the yogurt or labneh and a sprinkle of the mint.

Per serving: 395 calories, 31 g protein, 24 g carbohydrates, 2 g sugars, 21 g total fat, 4 g saturated fat, 6 g fiber, 462 mg sodium

189

Chapter 7
Dinner

Since folks in the Mediterranean enjoy their largest meal at lunch, it's common for dinner to be smaller and simpler. But it still tends to be an unhurried affair, where family members gather around the table to hang out, share stories, and just enjoy each other's company.

Of course, dinner tends to be the main meal of the day here at home—and for good reason. Even if you dedicate the time to a sit-down breakfast and lunch, it probably isn't until dinner that you get to kick back, relax, and catch up with the people you care about. So why not find ways to make those good feelings last a little longer?

Serving your dinner in courses, Mediterranean-style, can help you do just that. Though the mouthwatering dishes in this chapter are meant to be enjoyed as entrées, consider pairing them with the soups, salads, and sides in Chapters 5 and 6. Enjoying multiple dishes one by one is a simple way to stretch out your meal—plus it helps you eat slower and savor the taste of each individual dish. (For sample menu ideas, see page 276.) Here's how to do it.

• **SET OUT SOME LIGHT BITES.** Premeal snacks don't just whet the appetite—they encourage people to gather and relax before the meal even begins. And these sorts of nibbles don't have to be fussy. Try putting out a little bowl of olives or pickles, or a small plate of sliced raw vegetables with hummus, so everyone can nosh as the table gets set and the finishing touches get put on dinner.

• **START WITH A SALAD OR SOUP.** Some Medi-

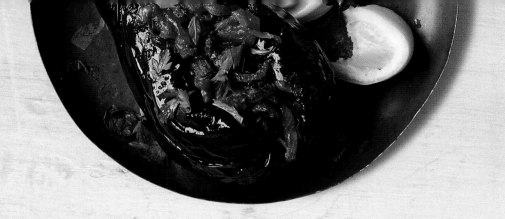

terranean cultures—like the Italians—save salad for the *end* of the meal, where it serves as a refreshing palate cleanser and digestive aid. But if you're making an effort to keep your portions in check, having those leafy greens before your main dish can help. In one study in the journal *Appetite*, participants ate 11 percent less of their pasta meal—and a whopping 23 percent more vegetables—when salad was served with it.[1] Findings show that starting with a bowl of broth-based soup can have a similar effect.[2]

• **TAKE A BREATHER BETWEEN BITES.** There's no rule that says you have to bring out the next course as soon as people have cleared their plates. If you're in the middle of a conversation—or just relishing the peace and quiet as you sit at the table—give your-self permission to stay put for a while. The food will still be there whenever you're ready to get up! Plus, pausing before adding more food to your plate will help you get a better handle on your fullness level. That can help you avoid overdoing it during the next course.

Recipes

OLIVE OIL–POACHED FISH OVER CITRUS SALAD

Poaching is a method of cooking that requires submerging the fish in a low-temperature liquid. The slow bath ensures even cooking and almost buttery results. This may seem like too much olive oil, but don't worry—it doesn't penetrate the fish, and barely a tablespoon clings to it when the fish is removed from the oil. While poaching can be done on a stove top, it requires a bit more monitoring to maintain the right heat. Instead, put this dish in the oven while you make the refreshing and bright citrus side salad. If wild salmon or Gulf shrimp are looking particularly appetizing at the fish market, feel free to substitute them here.

PREP TIME: 10 MINUTES / TOTAL TIME: 1 HOUR 15 MINUTES / SERVES 4

FISH

4	skinless white fish fillets (1¼–1½ pounds total), such as halibut, sole, or cod, ¾"–1" thick
¼	teaspoon kosher salt
¼	teaspoon ground black pepper
5–7	cups olive oil
1	lemon, thinly sliced

SALAD

¼	cup white wine vinegar
1	Earl Grey tea bag
2	blood oranges or tangerines
1	ruby red grapefruit or pomelo
6	kumquats, thinly sliced, or 2 clementines, peeled and sectioned
4	cups (4 ounces) baby arugula
½	cup pomegranate seeds
¼	cup extra-virgin olive oil
2	teaspoons minced shallot
½	teaspoon kosher salt
¼	teaspoon ground black pepper
¼	cup mint leaves, coarsely chopped

1. *To make the fish:* Season the fish with the salt and pepper and set aside for 30 minutes.

2. Preheat the oven to 225°F.

3. In a large high-sided ovenproof skillet or roasting pan over medium heat, warm 1" to 1½" of the oil and the lemon slices until the temperature reaches 120°F (use a candy thermometer). Add the fish fillets to the oil, without overlapping, making sure they're completely submerged.

4. Transfer the skillet or pan to the oven, uncovered. Bake for 25 minutes. Transfer the fish to a rack to drain for 5 minutes.

5. *To make the salad:* In a small saucepan, heat the vinegar until almost boiling. Add the tea bag and set aside to steep for 10 minutes.

(continued)

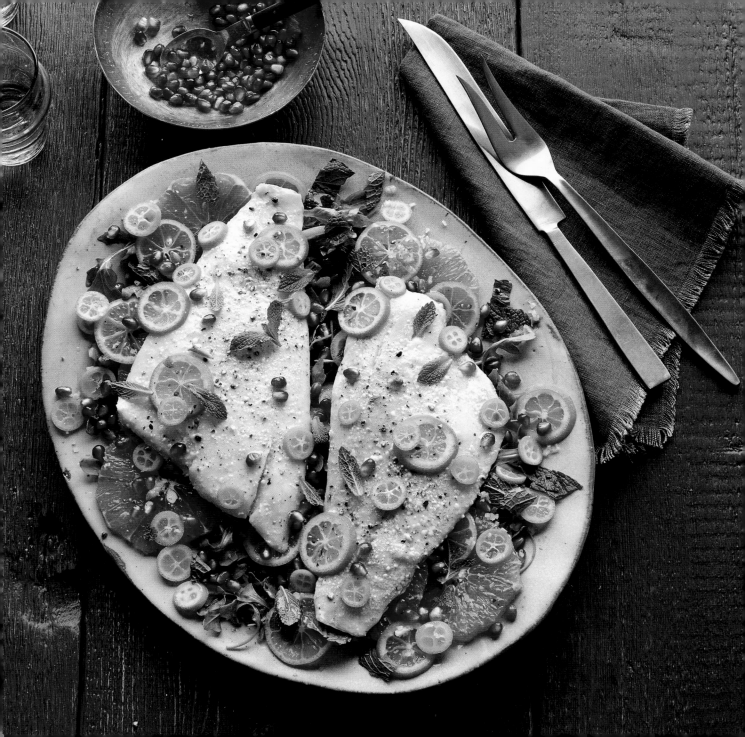

(continued from page 194)

6. Meanwhile, with a paring knife, cut off enough of the top and bottom of 1 of the oranges or tangerines to reveal the flesh. Cut along the inside of the peel, between the pith and the flesh, taking off as much pith as possible. Over a large bowl, hold the orange in 1 hand. With the paring knife, cut along the membranes between each section, allowing the fruit to fall into the bowl. Once all the fruit segments have been released, squeeze the remaining membranes over a small bowl. Repeat with the second orange and the grapefruit or pomelo.

7. In the large bowl with the segmented fruit, add the kumquats or clementines, arugula, and pomegranate seeds. Gently toss to distribute.

8. Remove the tea bag from the vinegar and squeeze out as much liquid as possible. Discard the bag and add the vinegar to the small bowl with the citrus juice. Slowly whisk in the oil, shallot, salt, and pepper. Drizzle 3 to 4 tablespoons over the salad and gently toss. (Store the remaining vinaigrette in the refrigerator for up to 1 week.)

9. Sprinkle the salad with the mint and serve with the fish.

Per serving: 280 calories, 29 g protein, 25 g carbohydrates, 17 g sugars, 7 g total fat, 1 g saturated fat, 6 g fiber, 249 mg sodium

LAMB KOFTA

These Middle Eastern–spiced meatballs are often served in a spicy tomato sauce or threaded onto skewers, as is done here.

PREP TIME: 15 MINUTES / TOTAL TIME: 25 MINUTES / SERVES 4

1   pound ground lamb
1   tablespoon chopped fresh mint
1½ teaspoons minced garlic (from 3 cloves), divided
2   teaspoons ground coriander
1   teaspoon ground cumin
1   teaspoon kosher salt
1–2 tablespoons olive oil
2   tablespoons low-fat plain Greek yogurt
2   tablespoons tahini
2   tablespoons fresh lemon juice

1. Coat a grill rack or grill pan with olive oil and prepare the grill to medium heat.

2. In a medium bowl, combine the lamb, mint, 1 teaspoon of the garlic, the coriander, cumin, and salt and mix until well blended. Divide into 8 balls and roll each ball into an elongated oval shape (like a football). Thread the meat onto metal skewers, 2 pieces per skewer, and brush with the oil.

3. Grill the skewers until cooked through and a thermometer inserted in the thickest part registers 160°F, turning once, 3 to 4 minutes per side.

4. In a small bowl, stir together the yogurt, tahini, lemon juice, and the remaining ½ teaspoon garlic. Serve the kofta with the sauce.

Per serving: 278 calories, 21 g protein, 4 g carbohydrate, 1 g sugars, 20 g total fat, 7 g saturated fat, 1 g fiber, 549 mg sodium

197

NOTE: This recipe works perfectly with Whole Wheat Pitas (page 164) or as part of a meze platter.

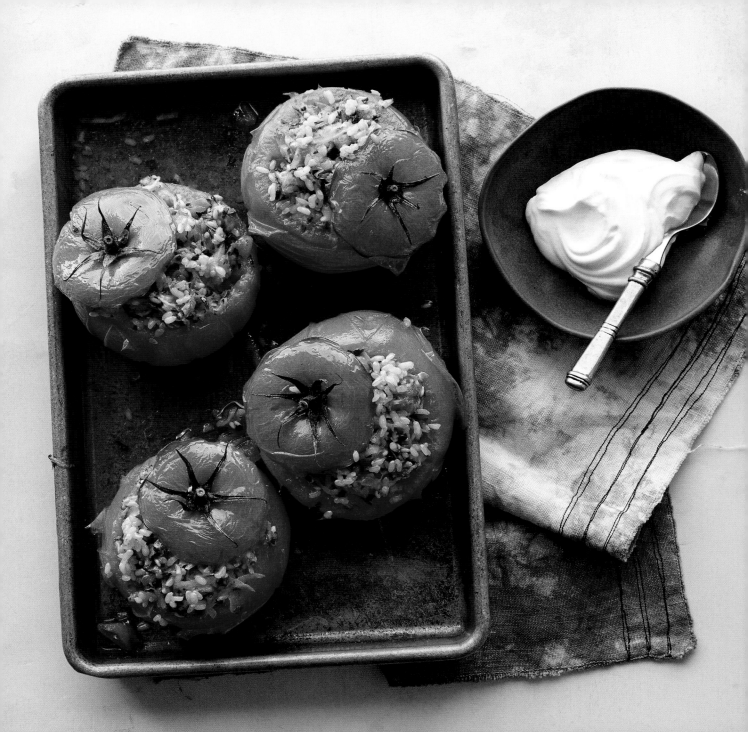

GEMISTA
(GREEK STUFFED TOMATOES)

To make preparing this dish a snap, use a grating blade on a food processor to prep your stuffing. To make this dish a complete dinner, go ahead and eat two!

PREP TIME: 20 MINUTES / TOTAL TIME: 2 HOURS / SERVES 10

10 large tomatoes
2   zucchini, grated
1   onion, grated
1   potato, grated
¾   cup short-grain brown rice
¼   cup chopped fresh flat-leaf parsley
2   tablespoons finely chopped fresh mint
1   tablespoon finely chopped fresh oregano
3   cloves garlic, minced
½   cup olive oil, divided
¼   cup fresh lemon juice
1   teaspoon kosher salt
½   teaspoon ground black pepper
1   cup water
1   cup low-fat plain Greek yogurt

1. Preheat the oven to 400°F.
2. Slice off ¼" from the top of the tomatoes with a serrated knife and set aside. Using a spoon, scoop out the tomato flesh and coarsely chop. Transfer to a large bowl. Place the tomatoes in a large baking dish.
3. In the large bowl with the tomato flesh, stir in the zucchini, onion, potato, rice, parsley, mint, oregano, and garlic. Add ¼ cup of the oil, the lemon juice, salt, and pepper and mix thoroughly.
4. Divide the filling among all the tomatoes, place the tops on them, and drizzle with the remaining ¼ cup oil. Pour the water into the baking dish and bake for 20 minutes.
5. Reduce the heat to 325°F, cover with foil, and continue baking until the rice is cooked through, about 1 hour, adding more water if the baking dish dries out.
6. Remove from the oven, remove the foil, and let the tomatoes sit for 10 minutes. Dollop with the yogurt before serving.

Per serving: 224 calories, 6 g protein, 26 g carbohydrates, 7 g sugars, 12 g total fat, 2 g saturated fat, 4 g fiber, 214 mg sodium

199

TOMATOES

Whether you call them a fruit or a vegetable, one thing's for sure: eating tomatoes Mediterranean-style is the healthiest way to enjoy them, since tomatoes cooked in olive oil have significantly more lycopene than their raw counterparts! A phytochemical thought to protect against prostate,[3] skin, breast, lung, and liver cancers, lycopene is a compound has also been shown to promote healthy blood vessel function and reduce the risk for stroke.[4]

SEARED SCALLOPS WITH BRAISED DANDELION GREENS

For an elegant dinner in just 20 minutes, serve these scallops with crusty whole grain bread and a glass of dry white wine.

PREP TIME: 5 MINUTES / TOTAL TIME: 20 MINUTES / SERVES 4

3   tablespoons olive oil, divided
2   cloves garlic, thinly sliced
1   pound dandelion greens
1   cup low-sodium chicken broth or water
½   teaspoon kosher salt, divided
¼   teaspoon ground black pepper, divided
1   cup chopped fresh mint
1   cup chopped fresh flat-leaf parsley
1   pound scallops, muscle tabs removed
     Lemon wedges, for serving

1. In a large skillet over medium-high heat, warm 1 tablespoon of the oil. Cook the garlic until softened, about 2 minutes. Add the dandelion greens and broth or water and bring to a boil. Cover and cook until the greens are wilted, 2 minutes. Season with ¼ teaspoon of the salt and ⅛ teaspoon of the pepper. Cover and cook until the greens are tender, 5 to 10 minutes. Stir in the mint and parsley.

2. Meanwhile, pat the scallops dry and season with the remaining ¼ teaspoon salt and the remaining ⅛ teaspoon pepper. In a large non-stick skillet over medium heat, warm 1 tablespoon of the oil. Add the scallops in a single layer and cook without disturbing until browned, 1 to 2 minutes. Add the remaining 1 tablespoon oil to the skillet, flip the scallops, and cook until browned on the other side, 1 to 2 minutes. Serve the scallops over the braised greens and with the lemon wedges.

Per serving: 235 calories, 18 g protein, 17 g carbohydrates, 1 g sugars, 12 g total fat, 2 g saturated fat, 5 g fiber, 850 mg sodium

200

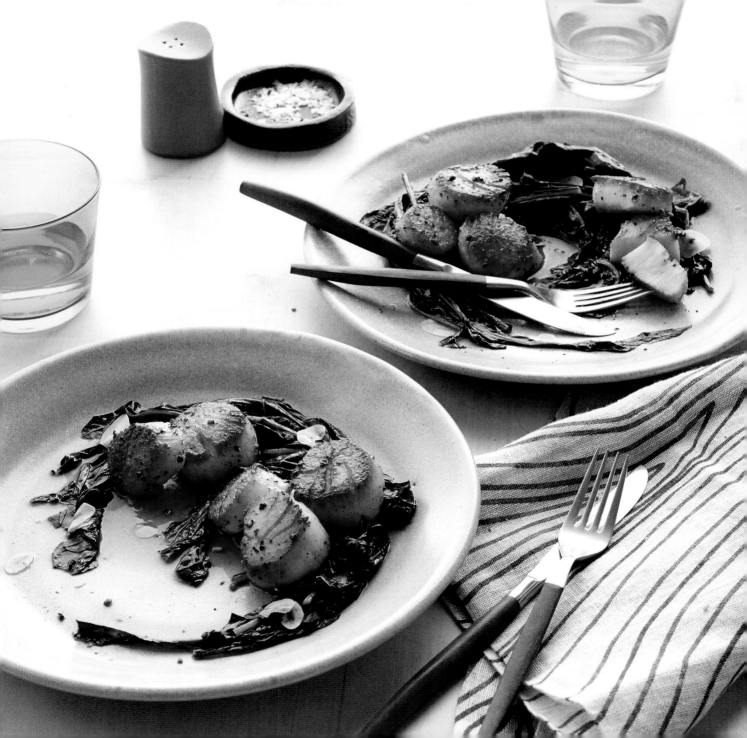

SLOW-COOKED PORK AND POTATOES

On Crete, trays of pork and potatoes are slow-roasted in traditional wood-burning ovens for hours to achieve meltingly tender results. Here, we transfer the dish to the slow cooker to similar effect.

PREP TIME: 15 MINUTES / TOTAL TIME: 8 HOURS 30 MINUTES / SERVES 8

- 1   teaspoon plus 2 tablespoons extra-virgin olive oil
- 2   pounds small red and yellow new potatoes, halved (quartered if large)
- 1   small white onion, thinly sliced
- 4   pounds boneless, skinless pork shoulder (Boston butt)
- 5   cloves garlic, minced
- 1   tablespoon chopped fresh oregano or 1 teaspoon dried
- 1   tablespoon chopped fresh rosemary or 1 teaspoon dried
- 1   tablespoon chopped fresh sage or 1 teaspoon dried
- 1   tablespoon chopped fresh thyme or 1 teaspoon dried
- 2   teaspoons kosher salt
- 1   teaspoon ground black pepper
- 1   cup low-sodium chicken broth

1. Brush the bottom of a 6-quart slow cooker with 1 teaspoon of the oil. Scatter the potatoes and onion on the bottom and place the pork on top. Using a sharp paring knife, poke holes throughout the entire pork shoulder.

2. In a small bowl, combine the remaining 2 tablespoons oil, the garlic, oregano, rosemary, sage, thyme, salt, and pepper. Pour over the pork. Using your fingers, poke some of the sauce into the holes. Pour in the broth around the pork. Cover and cook on low for about 8 hours or high for about 4 hours, occasionally turning the meat.

3. Remove the pork to a cutting board. Transfer the potatoes and onion to a serving platter and cover to keep warm.

4. Pour the juices from the slow cooker into a small saucepan and cook over medium-high heat until thickened and reduced, 8 to 10 minutes.

5. Break up the pork into large pieces and arrange on the platter with the potatoes. Pour the sauce over the pork or serve on the side.

Per serving: 300 calories, 28 g protein, 20 g carbohydrates, 2 g sugars, 12 g total fat, 3 g saturated fat, 2 g fiber, 595 mg sodium

202

ROASTED BRANZINO WITH FENNEL, LEMON, AND OLIVES

Save this for a dinner party or gathering: Serving the branzino whole makes for a grand presentation!

PREP TIME: 10 MINUTES / TOTAL TIME: 1 HOUR / SERVES 4

- 2 bulbs fennel, cored, wedged, and fronds reserved
- 1½ pounds baby potatoes, halved
- 1 lemon, sliced ¼" thick, divided
- ⅓ cup olive oil
- 3 tablespoons finely chopped fresh flat-leaf parsley
- 2 tablespoons finely chopped fresh dill
- Kosher salt and ground black pepper, to taste
- 2 pounds branzino (sea bass), cleaned with head and tail intact
- ½ cup pitted kalamata olives

1. Preheat the oven to 450°F.

2. In a large baking dish, add the fennel wedges, potatoes, and half of the lemon slices.

3. In a small bowl, combine the oil, parsley, and dill. Pour half the mixture over the vegetables, season with the salt and pepper to taste, and toss to combine. Roast the vegetables until beginning to brown, about 20 minutes.

4. Meanwhile, pat the fish dry and using a sharp knife, make 3 slashes along each side of flesh. Pour the other half of the oil mixture all over the fish, including inside the cavity. Season the fish all over with the salt and pepper to taste. Fill the cavity with the reserved fennel fronds and the remaining lemon slices.

5. Remove the baking dish from the oven and stir in the olives. Place the fish on top of the vegetables and return to the oven. Bake until the fish is opaque and the potatoes are tender, 20 minutes.

Per serving: 461 calories, 25 g protein, 31 g carbohydrates, 2 g sugars, 27 g total fat, 4 g saturated fat, 6 g fiber, 1,054 mg sodium

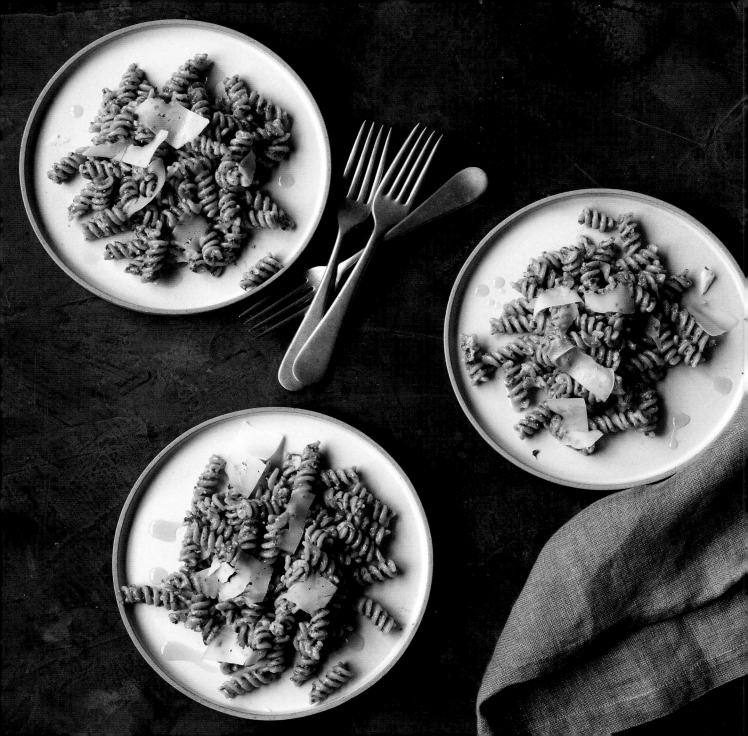

WHOLE WHEAT PASTA WITH ARUGULA-ALMOND PESTO

Nutty whole wheat pasta holds up well against the peppery flavors of this assertive pesto. To make this dish heartier, add a 15-ounce can of drained, rinsed chickpeas or white beans.

PREP TIME: 5 MINUTES / TOTAL TIME: 20 MINUTES / SERVES 6

1	pound whole wheat fusilli, rotini, or penne pasta
4	cups (4 ounces) baby arugula
¼	cup chopped raw almonds
1	clove garlic, minced
½	teaspoon kosher salt
¼	teaspoon ground black pepper
½	cup extra-virgin olive oil
1	ounce aged provolone cheese, grated

1. Cook the pasta according to package directions.

2. Meanwhile, in a food processor, pulse the arugula, almonds, garlic, salt, and pepper until coarsely chopped. Scrape down the sides of the bowl. With the processor running, stream in the oil. Stir in the cheese and put the pesto in a large serving bowl.

3. When the pasta is done, drain it and reserve a bit of the cooking water. Toss the pasta with the pesto, using the reserved pasta water if necessary to loosen the sauce.

Per serving: 451 calories, 12 g protein, 59 g carbohydrates, 3 g sugars, 19 g total fat, 3 g saturated fat, 8 g fiber, 253 mg sodium

205

PARCHMENT-BAKED HALIBUT WITH FENNEL AND CARROTS

Cooking foods in parchment paper, or *en papillote*, creates a small packet where the food is allowed to steam in its own juices. For a grand presentation, open them at the dinner table, where the herb-scented vapors will fill the room. Round out the meal with a light grain, such as whole wheat couscous.

PREP TIME: 10 MINUTES / TOTAL TIME: 35 MINUTES / SERVES 4

1   bulb fennel, cored, thinly sliced, and fronds reserved
1   bunch young carrots, quartered and tops removed
1   small shallot, sliced
4   skinless halibut fillets (6 ounces each)
½   teaspoon kosher salt
¼   teaspoon ground black pepper
4   slices orange
8   sprigs thyme
4   leaves fresh sage, sliced
½   cup white wine

1. Preheat the oven to 425°F. Tear 4 squares of parchment paper, about 15" x 15".

2. In the middle of a piece of parchment, set ¼ of the fennel, carrots, and shallot, topped by 1 piece of fish. Sprinkle with ⅛ teaspoon of the salt and a pinch of the pepper. Lay 1 slice of the orange, 2 sprigs of the thyme, ¼ of the sage, and a bit of fennel frond on top. Drizzle 2 tablespoons of the wine around the fish.

3. Bring up the opposite sides of the parchment and fold them together, like you're folding the top of a paper bag, to seal all the edges.

Set the packet on a baking sheet, and repeat with the remaining ingredients.

4. Bake until the packets are slightly browned and puffed, about 13 minutes. Allow to rest for 2 to 3 minutes. Set individual packets on plates and with kitchen shears or a small knife, carefully cut open at the table. (*Caution: The escaping steam will be hot.*)

Per serving: 253 calories, 34 g protein, 18 g carbohydrates, 6 g sugars, 3 g total fat, 0.5 g saturated fat, 5 g fiber, 455 mg sodium

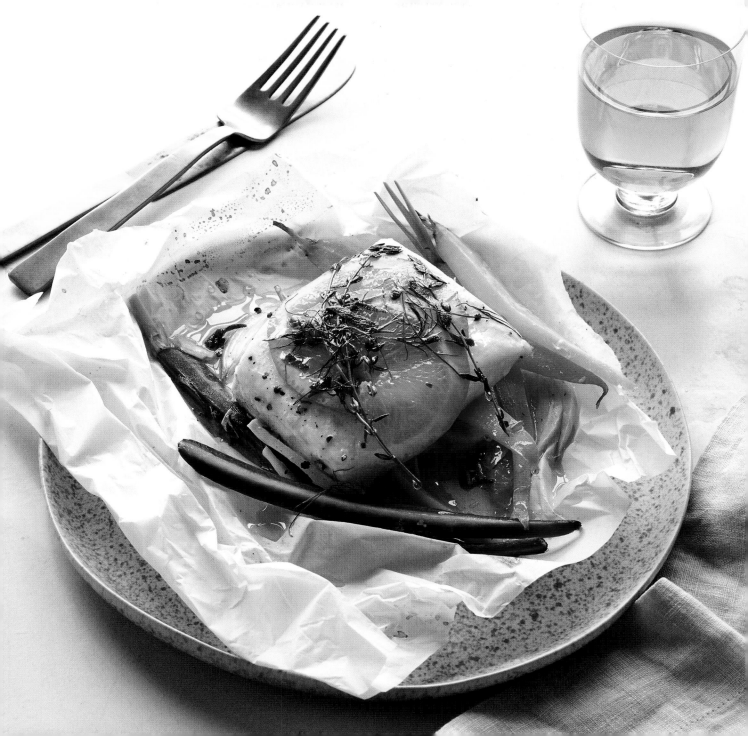

FARRO WITH ROASTED RED PEPPERS AND OLIVES

Salty feta and black olives complement the sweet, nutty farro and roasted red peppers in this warm grain salad.

PREP TIME: 5 MINUTES / TOTAL TIME: 30 MINUTES / SERVES 4

1	cup farro
3	tablespoons olive oil
1	tablespoon sherry vinegar
1	tablespoon honey
1	teaspoon chopped fresh thyme
1	clove garlic, mashed to a paste
½	teaspoon ground smoked paprika
¼	teaspoon kosher salt
2	roasted red peppers, coarsely chopped
½	cup crumbled feta
3	scallions, thinly sliced
¼	cup pitted black olives, slivered

1. Cook the farro according to package directions.

2. In a large bowl, whisk together the oil, vinegar, honey, thyme, garlic, paprika, and salt. Add the farro, peppers, cheese, scallions, and olives and toss well.

Per serving: 399 calories, 10 g protein, 45 g carbohydrates, 5 g sugars, 20 g total fat, 5 g saturated fat, 4 g fiber, 988 mg sodium

208

PAELLA

This classic Spanish seafood dish is traditionally served in a large, wide paella pan, into which everyone dips a fork to eat. The ingredients are inexpensive, and this dish adds an extra-special element to a festive dinner. We've included directions to transfer this recipe to 2 large skillets, but the recipe easily halves to fit into 1. The small amount of Spanish chorizo, a cooked sausage, adds just the right bit of smokiness to the rice, but feel free to leave it out.

PREP TIME: 25 MINUTES / TOTAL TIME: 2 HOURS / SERVES 8 TO 10

Generous pinch of saffron (about 20 threads)
20 large shrimp, peeled and deveined, shells reserved
8   cups water
4   bottles (8 ounces each) clam juice
⅓   cup extra-virgin olive oil
1   large white onion, diced
1   can (14.5 ounces) crushed tomatoes
2   links Spanish chorizo, diced
8   cloves garlic, minced
1   teaspoon mild or hot smoked Spanish paprika (pimenton)
¼   teaspoon kosher salt
¾   cup dry white wine
4   cups bomba rice
1   pound mussels, scrubbed and debearded (see note on page 103)
1   pound littleneck clams or pipis
¼   cup chopped fresh flat-leaf parsley
2   lemons, cut into wedges

1. In a 3-quart saucepan over medium heat, toast the saffron threads and shrimp shells, stirring often, until the shells are bright pink, about 2 minutes. Add the water and clam juice and bring to a boil. Turn off the heat and let steep. Strain before using (in Step 4) and discard the shrimp shells.

2. Meanwhile, in 2 large skillets or a 20" paella pan over medium heat, warm the oil. Cook the onion, stirring, until it softens and darkens slightly, about 5 minutes. Stir in the tomatoes, chorizo, garlic, paprika, and salt. Cook, stirring frequently, until deep red and thick, about 20 minutes. If it begins to stick before adding the wine, pour in little splashes of the wine to deglaze the pan.

3. Stir in the wine and cook until reduced and the mixture thickens to a paste, about 15 minutes. Adjust the heat as needed, being careful not to let the mixture burn.

(continued)

209

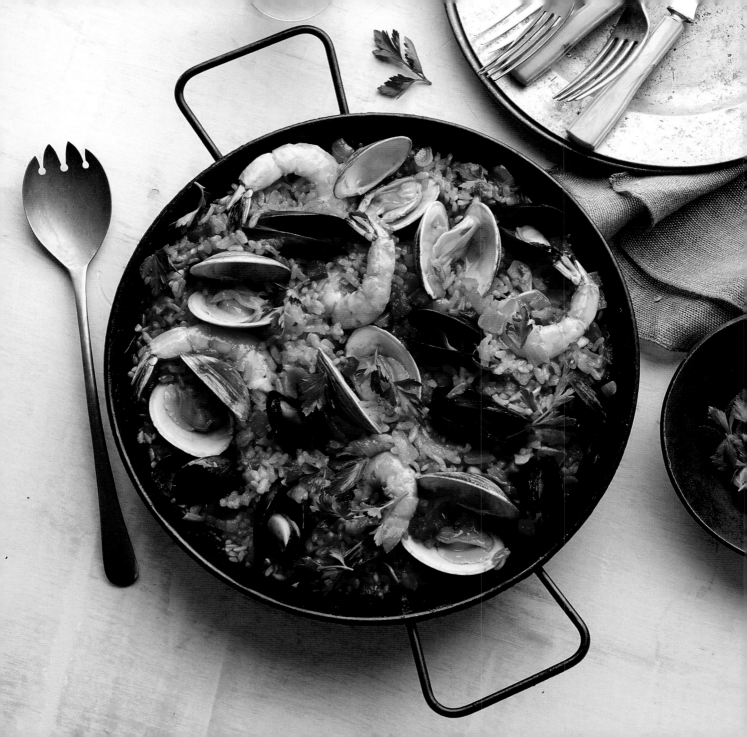

(continued from page 209)

4. Increase the heat to high. Add the rice and stir to combine, about 2 minutes. Spread the rice out evenly over the surface of the skillets or pan and gently pour in the saffron broth (6 cups per skillet, if using 2). Do not stir. Bring to a boil. Cook until the rice just begins to appear above the surface of the water, about 10 minutes.

5. Reduce the heat to maintain a simmer and push the mussels and clams into the rice. After 5 minutes, add the shrimp, pushing deep into the rice. Continue cooking until the rice is tender but still firm, about 10 minutes. Cover the skillets or pan with foil and cook 5 minutes.

6. Taste grains of rice from different parts of the pan to make sure it is cooked through. Use the tip of a spoon to check if the rice is caramelizing on the bottom. If the rice is cooked through, then increase the heat to medium-high, rotating the pan a bit to build up that delicious crispy bottom layer known as socarrat.

7. Remove the skillets or pan from the heat, cover with the foil, and let sit for 10 minutes. Remove any unopened shells, sprinkle with the parsley, and scatter the lemon wedges throughout. Gather your friends and family and eat your paella directly from the pan.

Per serving: 594 calories, 25 g protein, 88 g carbohydrates, 6 g fiber, 3 g sugars, 15 g total fat, 3 g saturated fat, 961 mg sodium

POLLO ALLA CALABRESE (CALABRIAN CHICKEN WITH POTATOES AND VEGETABLES)

Roasting the chicken, potatoes, and vegetables together makes this a convenient 1-pan meal from the Calabrian region of southwestern Italy.

PREP TIME: 10 MINUTES / TOTAL TIME: 1 HOUR / SERVES 4

4   chicken drumsticks
4   bone-in, skin-on chicken thighs
1   pint cherry tomatoes, halved
1   pound potatoes, scrubbed and cut into ½" wedges
3   red, orange, or yellow bell peppers, seeded and cut into ½" strips
1   large sweet onion, cut into ½" wedges
¼   cup olive oil
4   cloves garlic, minced
1   teaspoon dried oregano
1   teaspoon sweet paprika
1   teaspoon kosher salt
¼   teaspoon red-pepper flakes

1. Preheat the oven to 400°F.

2. On a large rimmed baking sheet, combine the chicken, tomatoes, potatoes, bell peppers, onion, oil, garlic, oregano, paprika, salt, and pepper flakes, tossing to combine and rubbing the chicken with the spices.

3. Arrange the vegetables underneath the chicken pieces. Roast until the vegetables are tender and a thermometer inserted in the thickest part of the chicken, but not touching bone, registers 165°F, about 45 minutes, turning the chicken and tossing the vegetables halfway through.

Per serving: 571 calories, 56 g protein, 34 g carbohydrates, 11 g sugars, 23 g total fat, 6 g saturated fat, 6 g fiber, 755 mg sodium

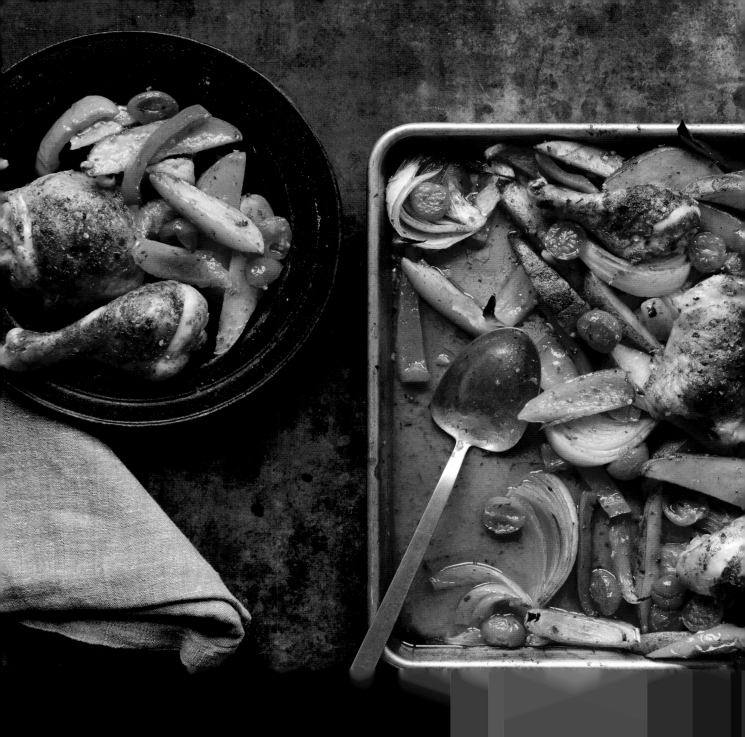

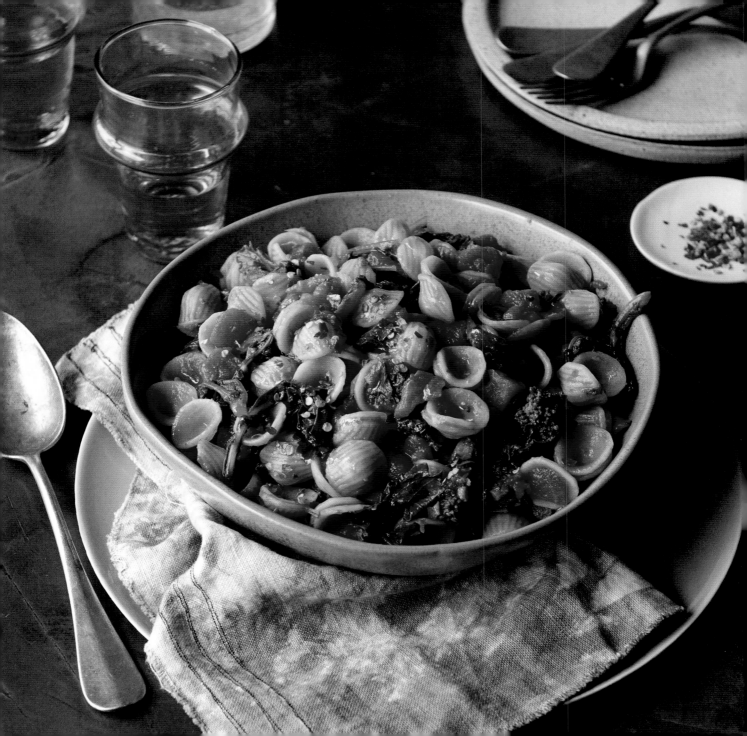

ORECCHIETTE WITH BROCCOLI RABE AND ANCHOVIES

Even if you're skeptical of anchovies, give this pasta dish a try. The anchovies practically melt into the warm olive oil, creating a pleasantly salty, savory flavor that isn't overly fishy.

PREP TIME: 5 MINUTES / TOTAL TIME: 25 MINUTES / SERVES 6

1   bunch broccoli rabe, chopped
1   pound whole wheat orecchiette pasta
¼   cup olive oil, divided
6   anchovy fillets, chopped
1   can (28 ounces) no-salt-added diced tomatoes
   Juice of 1 lemon
¼–½ teaspoon red-pepper flakes

1. Bring a large pot of salted water to a boil. Working in batches, plunge the broccoli rabe into the boiling water for 30 seconds. Using a slotted spoon, remove the broccoli rabe and transfer to a colander, drain, and set aside. Bring the pot of water back to a boil.

2. Add the pasta and cook according to package directions.

3. Meanwhile, in a large skillet over medium heat, warm 2 tablespoons of the oil and add the anchovies, breaking them up with a spoon. Add the tomatoes and cook to meld the flavors, 5 minutes. Add the broccoli rabe and stir.

4. When the pasta is done, drain and add to the skillet. Drizzle with the lemon juice and the remaining 2 tablespoons oil and toss gently. Sprinkle with pepper flakes and serve.

Per serving: 426 calories, 14 g protein, 67 g carbohydrates, 8 g sugars, 11 g total fat, 1.5 g saturated fat, 8 g fiber, 198 mg sodium

FATTY FISH

Here's a startling stat: Eating one to two 3-ounce servings of fatty fish per week could reduce the risk of dying from heart disease by a whopping 36 percent, found a major *JAMA* analysis of 20 studies.[5] The essential omega-3 fatty acids found in fish like salmon, mackerel, herring, anchovies, and sardines help lower blood pressure and heart rate, promote healthy blood vessel function, fight unhealthy levels of fat in the blood, and reduce inflammation. ("Essential" means that the body doesn't produce these nutrients on its own; you need to get them from food.)

Heart health isn't the only thing that makes fatty fish a great catch. The body needs omega-3s to regulate genetic function (when cells produce more or less of certain genetic materials) and to produce hormones that keep inflammation in check. Likely, that's why these important fats have also been shown to protect against cancer and Alzheimer's disease, as well as help manage chronic conditions like eczema and rheumatoid arthritis. They might even improve your mood. Though more research is needed, some findings suggest that omega-3 fatty acids could be beneficial for adults with mild to moderate depression.[6]

Still, fish contains contaminants like mercury and polychlorinated biphenyls (PCBs)—which could be harmful in high doses. So is it safe to serve seafood on a regular basis? The answer is a resounding yes, experts say. The massive health benefits that come with eating fatty fish far outweigh any potential health risks, especially when you make the effort to eat a wide variety of fish and seafood. So grab your fork and dive in. The water's just fine!

216

KUSHARI
(EGYPTIAN RICE, LENTILS, AND DITALINI)

Kushari is considered one of Egypt's most well-known dishes and is very popular at roadside stands and eateries all over the country. You can spice it up by adding hot sauce or a sprinkle of red-pepper flakes, if you like. We love to make a double batch of the sliced onions and put them on everything.

PREP TIME: 5 MINUTES / TOTAL TIME: 35 MINUTES / SERVES 8

- 8 ounces ditalini pasta
- 1 cup French green lentils, rinsed
- 3 tablespoons olive oil, divided
- 2 yellow onions, 1½ very thinly sliced, ½ coarsely chopped
- 6 cloves garlic, minced
- 2 cups tomato puree
- 1 teaspoon ground cumin
- ½ teaspoon kosher salt
- ¼ teaspoon ground black pepper
- ¼ teaspoon chili powder
- ⅛ teaspoon ground cinnamon
- 1 tablespoon apple cider vinegar
- 2 cups cooked brown rice
- 1 cup drained and rinsed canned chickpeas

1. Cook the pasta according to package directions. Drain and set aside. Cook the lentils according to package directions. Drain and set aside.

2. Meanwhile, in a medium skillet over medium-low heat, warm 2 tablespoons of the oil. Cook the onion slices, stirring often, until very soft and browned, 30 minutes.

3. While the sliced onions are cooking, in a medium saucepan over medium heat, warm the remaining 1 tablespoon oil. Cook the coarsely chopped onion until softened, 5 minutes. Add the garlic and cook 1 minute. Add the tomato puree, cumin, salt, pepper, chili powder, and cinnamon. Stir to combine, cover, and simmer to meld the flavors, 10 minutes. Stir in the vinegar.

4. To assemble, mix together the pasta, lentils, brown rice, and chickpeas. Serve topped with the tomato sauce and the caramelized onions.

Per serving: 351 calories, 13 g protein, 61 g carbohydrates, 7 g sugars, 7 g total fat, 1 g saturated fat, 9 g fiber, 403 mg sodium

217

LAMB AND ONION TAGINE

Serve this rich lamb tagine as it might be served in Morocco—with whole wheat couscous to soak up all of the flavorful juices.

PREP TIME: 10 MINUTES / TOTAL TIME: 3 HOURS 35 MINUTES / SERVES 4

- 2 tablespoons finely chopped fresh flat-leaf parsley
- 2 tablespoons finely chopped fresh cilantro
- 2 cloves garlic, minced
- ½ teaspoon ground turmeric
- ½ teaspoon ground ginger
- 1 teaspoon ground cinnamon, divided
- 1 teaspoon plus a pinch kosher salt
- ½ teaspoon ground black pepper
- 2 tablespoons plus ⅓ cup water
- 3 tablespoons extra-virgin olive oil
- 4 bone-in leg of lamb steaks, ½" thick (about 2½ pounds)
- 1 can (28 ounces) whole peeled plum tomatoes, drained
- 2 large red onions, 1 finely chopped, the other sliced in ⅛" rounds
- 2 teaspoons honey, divided
- 1 tablespoon toasted sesame seeds

1. In a large bowl, combine the parsley, cilantro, garlic, turmeric, ginger, ¼ teaspoon of the cinnamon, 1 teaspoon of the salt, and the pepper. Add 2 tablespoons of the water and the oil and mix. Add the lamb steaks and turn to coat each one. Cover and refrigerate, turning the steaks occasionally, for at least 1 hour.

2. Make a small cut into each tomato and squeeze out the seeds and excess juices.

3. In a 12" tagine or a deep heavy-bottom skillet, scatter the chopped onion. Arrange the lamb steaks snugly in a single layer. Drizzle the remaining marinade over the top. Add the tomatoes around the lamb. Drizzle 1 teaspoon of the honey and ¼ teaspoon of the cinnamon over the top.

4. Lay the onion rounds on top of the lamb. Drizzle the remaining 1 teaspoon honey. Sprinkle the remaining ½ teaspoon cinnamon and the pinch of salt. Turn the heat on to medium (medium-low if using a pot) and cook, uncovered, nudging the lamb occasionally, until the chopped onion below is translucent, about 15 minutes.

5. Pour in the ⅓ cup water around the outer edges of the food. Cover with a lid, slightly askew to keep air flowing in and out of the tagine or skillet. Reduce the heat to low and simmer gently, nudging the lamb occasionally to prevent sticking. Cook until the lamb is very tender, adding water as needed to keep the sauce moist, about 2 hours.

6. Sprinkle with the sesame seeds and serve.

Per serving: 448 calories, 44 g protein, 16 g carbohydrates, 9 g sugars, 23 g total fat, 6 g saturated fat, 3 g fiber, 913 mg sodium

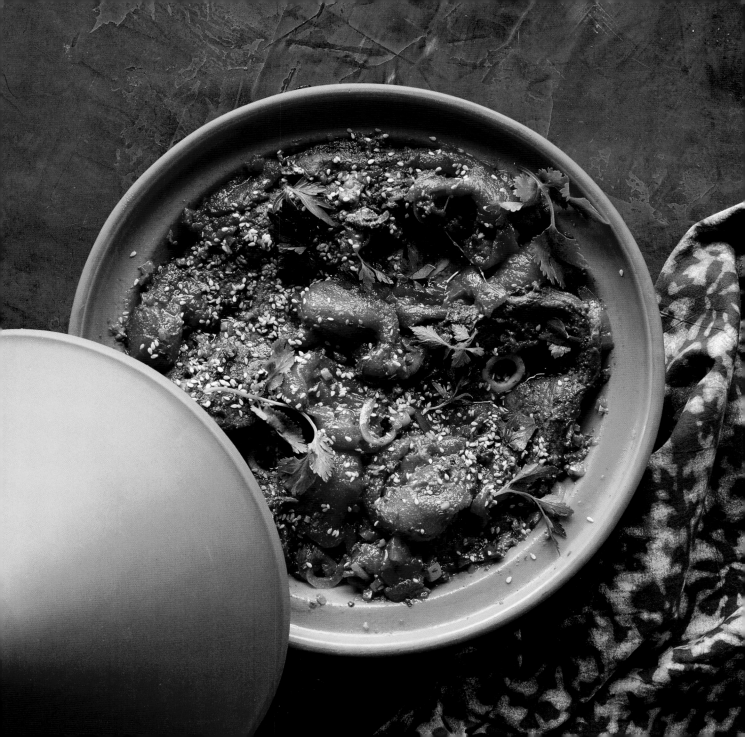

VEGETARIAN MOUSSAKA

This Greek casserole is typically layered with zucchini, eggplant, tomatoes, and potatoes—sometimes with ground meat, sometimes without. It's like lasagna without the noodles. Traditionally slathered with a rich béchamel sauce—cream thickened with butter and flour—we've lightened up this meatless version in more ways than one. While rustic, this dish definitely takes time, patience, and a little love to prepare. The good news is that portions freeze well so you can have comfort food any time. The moussaka may even be assembled through Step 13, then refrigerated for 1 day covered, and set out for 1 hour before baking. Simply increase the bake time by 10 minutes to compensate for the cold and get the center hot.

PREP TIME: 25 MINUTES / TOTAL TIME: 3 HOURS 30 MINUTES / SERVES 8 TO 12

½ ounce dried porcini mushrooms
1 cup boiling water
1 yellow onion, thinly sliced
4 tablespoons olive oil, divided
8 ounces sliced fresh cremini mushrooms
2 cloves garlic, sliced
1 bay leaf
2 teaspoons dried oregano
1 teaspoon kosher salt, divided, plus more for eggplant
1 teaspoon ground black pepper, divided
½ teaspoon ground cinnamon
¼ teaspoon ground nutmeg
  Pinch of ground cloves
1 cup dry red wine
2 cans (15 ounces each) chickpeas, drained and rinsed (see note on page 80)
2 cans (14.5 ounces each) diced fire-roasted tomatoes
½ cup brown lentils, rinsed
1 large eggplant (1½–2 pounds), sliced lengthwise ¼" thick (see note opposite)

2 pounds russet potatoes, peeled and coarsely chopped
¾ cup low-fat plain Greek yogurt
2 eggs, beaten
½ cup part-skim ricotta cheese
2 ounces feta cheese, finely crumbled
2 zucchini, sliced lengthwise ¼" thick

1. In a small bowl, cover the porcini mushrooms with the boiling water and set aside to soak for 10 minutes. Remove the mushrooms (save the water) and coarsely chop.

2. Meanwhile, in a very large skillet over medium heat, cook the onion in 1 tablespoon of the oil until softened, 5 minutes. Add the cremini mushrooms and cook until their liquid is nearly all out, about 5 minutes. Add the porcini mushrooms and garlic and cook, stir-

ring frequently, until the liquid is nearly evaporated, 2 minutes more.

3. Add the bay leaf, oregano, ½ teaspoon each of the salt and pepper, the cinnamon, nutmeg, and cloves. Cook, stirring constantly, for 1 minute.

4. Add the wine and reduce, scraping the bottom of the skillet, until the skillet is nearly dry, 5 to 8 minutes.

5. Add the chickpeas, tomatoes, and lentils. Slowly pour the reserved mushroom water into the skillet, leaving the dirt and silt at the bottom of the bowl. Thoroughly stir the mixture.

6. Increase the heat to medium-high and bring to a boil. Reduce the heat to medium-low and keep at a bare simmer, stirring occasionally, until the lentils are tender and the sauce is quite thick and nearly dry, 45 minutes. Remove the bay leaf.

7. Meanwhile, put the eggplant in a colander and sprinkle with a good pinch of the salt. Set aside to drain for 30 minutes. Rinse the eggplant and pat dry with paper towels.

8. While the eggplant is draining, put the potatoes in a large saucepan and cover with 1" of lightly salted water. Bring to a boil and cook until the potatoes are very tender, 15 to 20 minutes. Drain and return the potatoes to the saucepan and stir over medium-low heat for 1 minute.

221

(continued)

(continued from page 221)

9. Remove the potatoes from the heat and add the yogurt, eggs, ricotta, feta, and the remaining ½ teaspoon each salt and pepper. Mash until desired consistency.

10. Turn the oven on to broil and set a rack 6" from the heat. Brush a large baking sheet with 1 teaspoon of the oil. Set the eggplant slices on the sheet and brush with 1 tablespoon of the oil. Broil until golden and slightly charred in places, turning over the slices once, about 5 minutes total. Transfer to a rack. Repeat this step with the zucchini.

11. Preheat the oven to 350°F.

12. Brush a deep 9" x 13" baking dish with the remaining 1 teaspoon oil. Spread 2 cups of the chickpea mixture in the bottom. Top with a layer of eggplant, followed by a layer of zucchini. Spread 2 to 3 cups of the chickpea mixture over the zucchini. Repeat layering once more, ending with the remaining chickpea mixture.

13. Spread the potato mixture over the top, covering the chickpea mixture completely.

14. Bake until the potatoes are golden and the eggplant and zucchini are tender, 30 to 45 minutes. Rest at least 20 minutes before slicing and serving.

Per serving: 421 calories, 19 g protein, 55 g carbohydrates, 11 g sugars, 13 g total fat, 4 g saturated fat, 12 g fiber, 861 mg sodium

RED WINE

And now, a toast to one of the world's healthiest drinks. Enjoying moderate amounts of red wine is linked to a host of impressive benefits, including a lower risk for heart disease, Alzheimer's disease, depression, and even certain cancers. The benefits are thought to come from resveratrol, a polyphenol that promotes healthy blood vessels and also fights the buildup of LDL, or "bad," cholesterol. That's not the only good-for-you compound you'll get from a glass of vino, though. Red wine also serves up procyanidins, a group of flavonoids thought to play a role in longevity in a study of moderate wine drinkers in the Mediterranean regions of Sardinia and southwest France.[7]

Of course, if you choose to drink, a middle-of-the-road approach is best. Consuming too much alcohol can increase your chances for heart disease, obesity, high blood pressure, stroke, and cancer. So how much *should* you have? According to one *Annals of Internal Medicine* study, one 5-ounce glass per day might be the magic number.[8] Subjects with controlled type 2 diabetes were randomly assigned to have that much red wine, white wine, or mineral water with dinner each night. Over the 2-year study period, red wine drinkers increased their HDL, or "good," cholesterol, showed fewer components of metabolic syndrome, and even slept better than the mineral water drinkers.

Make it a point to sip your wine with a meal, rather than by itself. Having a glass of wine with dinner (or lunch, if you'd prefer) encourages you to take a break in between bites and relax at the table, while food helps slow the absorption of alcohol. And though culinary custom might dictate enjoying seafood with white wine, consider pairing it with red instead. Studies suggest that it may boost the absorption of the omega-3 fatty acids found in fish like salmon.[9] *Salud!*

223

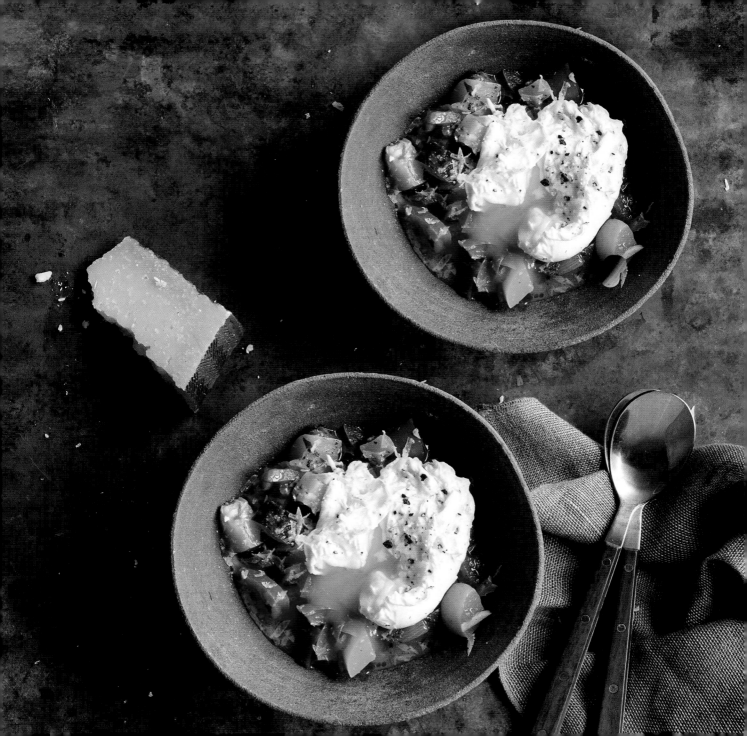

PISTO WITH POACHED EGGS AND MANCHEGO
(SPANISH RATATOUILLE)

You might associate eggs with breakfast. But in Spain, pisto topped with the traditional poached egg—which comes from the region of La Mancha—is often eaten at lunch or dinner with fresh bread.

PREP TIME: 15 MINUTES / TOTAL TIME: 1 HOUR / SERVES 4

¼ cup extra-virgin olive oil, preferably Spanish, divided
1 Spanish onion, diced
3 cloves garlic, minced
½ teaspoon ground cumin
1 large red bell pepper, seeded and diced
1 small green bell pepper, seeded and diced
1 small zucchini, diced
1 small yellow squash, diced
½ cup dry sherry or white wine
8 plum tomatoes, diced
4 eggs
3 tablespoons finely chopped fresh flat-leaf parsley
1 tablespoon sherry vinegar
Kosher salt and ground black pepper, to taste
¼ cup finely grated aged Manchego cheese

1. In a large skillet over medium heat, warm 2 tablespoons of the oil until shimmering. Cook the onion and garlic, stirring, until the onion is translucent, about 8 minutes. Stir in the cumin and cook until fragrant, about 1 minute.

2. Add the bell peppers, zucchini, and squash and cook until the zucchini and squash soften, about 5 minutes. Pour in the sherry or wine, bring to a simmer, and cook until reduced to 2 tablespoons, about 5 minutes.

3. Stir in the tomatoes and reduce the heat to low. Cook until the vegetables are completely tender and the juices have evaporated, about 30 minutes.

4. Meanwhile, bring a medium pot of water to a simmer. Using a slotted spoon, swirl the water like a whirlpool. Add each egg individually, making sure they don't land on each other. Cook until the whites are firm but not hard, 3 to 5 minutes.

5. In the large skillet, stir in the parsley, vinegar, and the remaining 2 tablespoons oil and season to taste with the salt and black pepper. Divide the vegetables among 4 shallow bowls. Top each with an egg and a sprinkling of the cheese.

Per serving: 364 calories, 14 g protein, 18 g carbohydrates, 10 g sugars, 25 g total fat, 7 g saturated fat, 5 g fiber, 453 mg sodium

FETTUCCINE WITH SPICY GARLICKY DANDELION GREENS

Italian cooks know that the secret to a velvety pasta sauce is in the pasta cooking water: The starch leftover from the pasta acts as a thickener, so you don't need to use a heavy hand with rich ingredients like oil, cream, or cheese.

PREP TIME: 10 MINUTES / TOTAL TIME: 30 MINUTES / SERVES 6

1 pound whole wheat fettuccine
¼ cup olive oil
3 cloves garlic, thinly sliced
¼ teaspoon red-pepper flakes, plus more for serving
2 large bunches dandelion greens, trimmed and coarsely chopped
½ teaspoon kosher salt, plus more to taste
⅔ cup finely grated Parmigiano-Reggiano cheese, plus more for serving
1 tablespoon lemon juice
1½ teaspoons grated lemon peel

1. Cook the fettuccine according to package directions.

2. Meanwhile, in a large skillet over medium heat, cook the oil, garlic, and pepper flakes until the garlic begins to turn golden, about 2 minutes. Add the greens and salt and toss in the oil until completely coated. Cover and cook, tossing occasionally, until the greens are wilted, about 2 minutes.

3. When the pasta is done, drain it and reserve 1 cup of the cooking water. Toss the pasta in with the greens. Add the cheese and toss to incorporate, adding a bit of the pasta water to keep the mixture moist.

4. Season to taste with the salt and add the lemon juice. Top with more cheese and pepper flakes and the lemon peel.

Per serving: 467 calories, 21 g protein, 71 g carbohydrates, 4 g sugars, 15 g total fat, 3.5 g saturated fat, 14 g fiber, 504 mg sodium

226

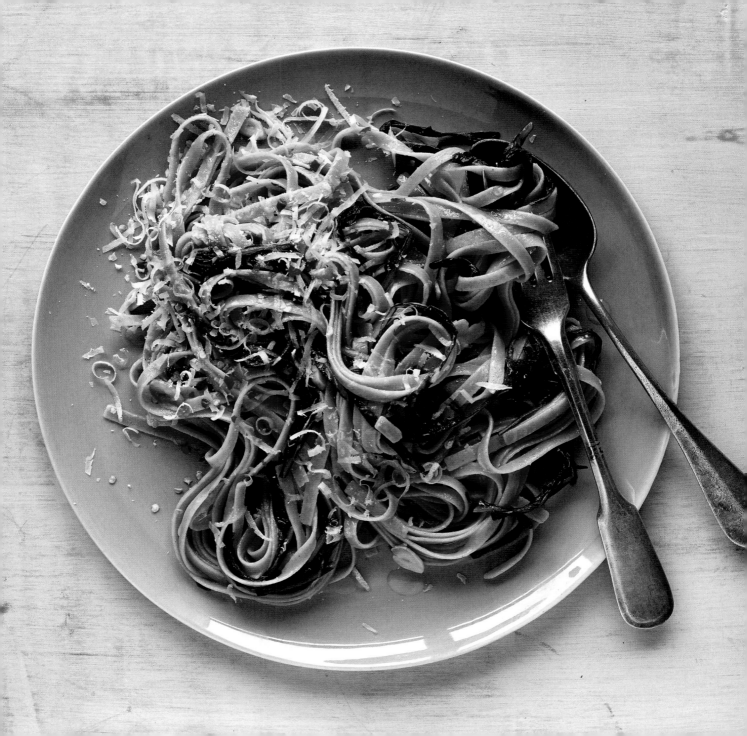

PORK TENDERLOIN WITH BRUSSELS SPROUTS AND PEARL ONIONS

Pork gets the Mediterranean treatment with fresh rosemary, which adds a fresh, piney flavor to this hearty dish.

PREP TIME: 5 MINUTES / TOTAL TIME: 45 MINUTES / SERVES 4

1 pork tenderloin (about 1 pound), trimmed
2 tablespoons olive oil, divided
½ teaspoon kosher salt
¼ teaspoon ground black pepper
2 cups frozen and thawed peeled pearl onions
2 cups Brussels sprouts, halved
2 or 3 sprigs fresh rosemary
1 cup red wine or low-sodium chicken broth

1. Preheat the oven to 400°F.

2. Pat the tenderloin dry, rub with 1 tablespoon of the oil, and sprinkle with the salt and pepper. In a large ovenproof skillet over medium heat, sear the tenderloin on all sides until browned, about 3 minutes per side. Remove from the heat and set aside.

3. Toss the onions, Brussels sprouts, and rosemary with the remaining 1 tablespoon oil in the skillet. Place the tenderloin on top of the vegetables and herbs and roast until a thermometer placed in the thickest part reaches 145°F, about 15 minutes. Remove the skillet from the oven and transfer the tenderloin and vegetables to a serving plate to rest while you make the sauce.

4. On the stove top, add the wine or broth to the skillet and bring to a boil, scraping up any browned bits on the bottom of the skillet. Cook until reduced and slightly thickened, 10 to 15 minutes. Remove the rosemary sprigs. Slice the tenderloin and serve with the vegetables and sauce.

Per serving: 310 calories, 27 g protein, 20 g carbohydrates, 5 g sugars, 9 g total fat, 2 g saturated fat, 2 g fiber, 380 mg sodium (with wine) or 397 mg (with broth)

228

FABADA
(SPANISH HAM STEW)

Though this Spanish-style stew has its origins in the northwestern region of Asturias, it can be found in many incarnations all over Spain. It generally includes a cured form of pork. Here, we've lightened it up with leaner ham and added smokiness and depth with smoked paprika.

PREP TIME: 15 MINUTES / TOTAL TIME: 50 MINUTES / SERVES 4 TO 6

1 tablespoon olive oil
1 boneless ham steak (8 ounces), diced
1 onion, finely chopped
1 tablespoon tomato paste
1 tablespoon smoked paprika
1 bay leaf
1 teaspoon dried rosemary
1 clove garlic, minced
3 cups low-sodium chicken broth
1 sweet potato, peeled and cut into ½" cubes
1 can (15 ounces) white beans (cannellini beans, great Northern beans, butter beans), drained and rinsed (see note on page 80)
¼ cup chopped fresh flat-leaf parsley
¼ cup slivered almonds

1. In a 4-quart saucepan or Dutch oven over medium heat, warm the oil. Cook the ham and onion, stirring occasionally, until the onion is tender, 5 minutes. Add the tomato paste, paprika, bay leaf, rosemary, and garlic and cook, stirring constantly, 1 minute.

2. Add the broth, sweet potato, and beans and bring to a boil. Reduce the heat to medium-low and simmer until the sweet potato is tender, about 20 minutes.

3. Meanwhile, in a small skillet over medium heat, toast the almonds, 5 minutes. Remove the almonds from the skillet to cool.

4. Remove the bay leaf. Stir in the parsley before serving. Top with the almonds.

Per serving: 298 calories, 23 g protein, 29 g carbohydrates, 4 g sugars, 11 g total fat, 2 g saturated fat, 6 g fiber, 823 mg sodium

MEDITERRANEAN SPICE-CRUSTED SALMON OVER WHITE BEANS

This Italian-inspired salmon feels elegant and special—but it's ready in just about half an hour.

PREP TIME: 10 MINUTES / TOTAL TIME: 35 MINUTES / SERVES 6

¼ cup olive oil, divided
1 large bulb fennel, cored and thinly sliced
1 yellow onion, diced
2 cloves garlic, minced
½ cup white wine
3 cans (15 ounces each) no-salt-added cannellini beans, drained and rinsed (see note on page 80)
1 can (14.5 ounces) diced fire-roasted tomatoes
1 teaspoon Dijon mustard
⅛ teaspoon red-pepper flakes
1 tablespoon fennel seeds
2 teaspoons ground black pepper
1 teaspoon kosher salt
6 wild salmon fillets (6 ounces each)
¼ cup thinly sliced basil

1. In a large skillet over medium heat, warm 2 tablespoons of the oil until shimmering. Cook the sliced fennel, onion, and garlic, stirring, until tender, about 8 minutes. Stir in the wine and cook until reduced by half, about 5 minutes. Add the beans and tomatoes and cook, stirring occasionally, to meld all the flavors, about 10 minutes. Stir in the mustard and pepper flakes.

2. Meanwhile, in a small bowl, combine the fennel seeds, black pepper, and salt. Sprinkle all over the salmon fillets.

3. In a large nonstick skillet over medium heat, warm the remaining 2 tablespoons oil. Cook the salmon, skin side up, until golden brown, about 5 minutes. Flip and cook until your desired doneness, about 3 minutes for medium.

4. Stir the basil into the bean mixture just before serving, divide among 6 shallow bowls, and top each with a salmon fillet.

Per serving: 488 calories, 42 g protein, 30 g carbohydrates, 4 g sugars, 22 g total fat, 3 g saturated fat, 9 g fiber, 745 mg sodium

GRILLED ROSEMARY-LEMON TURKEY CUTLETS

Marinating turkey in rosemary before grilling isn't just delicious: The herb's antioxidant compounds have been shown to significantly reduce the formation of heterocyclic amines (HCAs)—carcinogenic compounds that form when meat or poultry is cooked at a high temperature.[10]

PREP TIME: 10 MINUTES / TOTAL TIME: 40 MINUTES / SERVES 4

2 tablespoons olive oil
2 tablespoons fresh lemon juice
1 teaspoon finely chopped fresh rosemary
1 clove garlic, minced
4 turkey cutlets (6 ounces each), pounded to ¼" thickness
  Kosher salt and ground black pepper, to taste
2 ripe tomatoes, diced
½ red onion, diced
1 tablespoon balsamic vinegar
2 cups (2 ounces) baby arugula

1. In a large bowl, combine the oil, lemon juice, rosemary, and garlic. Add the turkey cutlets and let marinate at room temperature while you prepare the grill, about 20 minutes.

2. Coat a grill rack or grill pan with olive oil and prepare the grill to medium-high heat.

3. Season the turkey with the salt and pepper. Grill the cutlets until grill marks form and the turkey is cooked through, about 4 minutes per side.

4. Meanwhile, in a medium bowl, combine the tomatoes, onion, and vinegar and season to taste with the salt and pepper.

5. Top each cutlet with ½ cup baby arugula and a quarter of the tomato mixture.

Per serving: 269 calories, 43 g protein, 6 g carbohydrates, 3 g sugars, 8 g total fat, 1 g saturated fat, 1 g fiber, 398 mg sodium

231

MUSHROOM RAGU WITH POLENTA

A combination of fresh and dried mushrooms packs loads of savory flavor into this hearty dish. It's vegetarian if you use vegetable broth, and to make it vegan, simply omit the Parmigiano-Reggiano cheese.

PREP TIME: 15 MINUTES / TOTAL TIME: 45 MINUTES / SERVES 4

½   ounce dried porcini mushrooms
2   cups hot water
2   cups water
1   cup polenta
1   teaspoon kosher salt, divided
¼   cup grated Parmigiano-Reggiano cheese
1   tablespoon olive oil
2   shallots, chopped
1   pound fresh mushrooms, such as white, shiitake, oyster, cremini, or a mix, coarsely chopped
1   teaspoon chopped fresh rosemary
¼   teaspoon ground black pepper
2   teaspoons all-purpose flour
1   cup low-sodium chicken broth or vegetable broth

1. In a medium bowl, add the porcini mushrooms and hot water. Let them soak for 15 minutes, and then remove the mushrooms and coarsely chop. Reserve the soaking water.

2. In a medium saucepan, bring the water and the reserved mushroom soaking water (leaving any silt behind in the bowl) to a boil. Add the polenta and ½ teaspoon of the salt, lower the heat to a simmer, and cook, stirring frequently, until thickened and smooth, about 30 minutes. Stir in the cheese.

3. Meanwhile, in a large skillet over medium heat, warm the oil. Cook the shallots until softened, about 5 minutes. Add the porcini mushrooms, fresh mushrooms, rosemary, pepper, and the remaining ½ teaspoon salt. Cook until the mushrooms release their liquid and soften, about 5 minutes. Add the flour and stir until incorporated. Add the broth, increase the heat, and bring to a boil. Reduce the heat to a simmer and cook until the liquid is reduced and thickened, 10 to 15 minutes.

4. To serve, mound the polenta in a wide shallow bowl and top with the mushroom ragu.

Per serving: 235 calories, 11 g protein, 37 g carbohydrates, 4 g sugars, 6 g total fat, 1.5 g saturated fat, 4 g fiber, 700 mg sodium

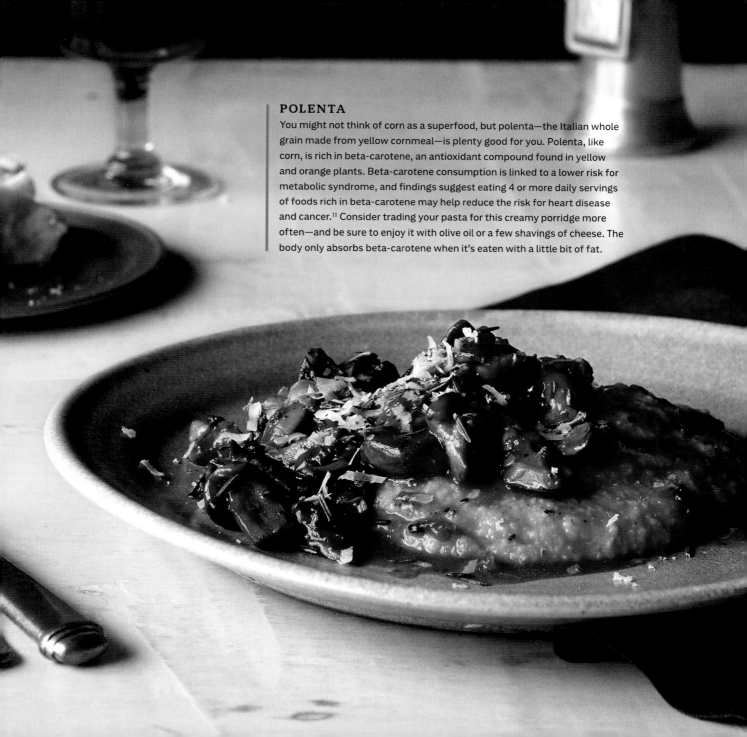

POLENTA

You might not think of corn as a superfood, but polenta—the Italian whole grain made from yellow cornmeal—is plenty good for you. Polenta, like corn, is rich in beta-carotene, an antioxidant compound found in yellow and orange plants. Beta-carotene consumption is linked to a lower risk for metabolic syndrome, and findings suggest eating 4 or more daily servings of foods rich in beta-carotene may help reduce the risk for heart disease and cancer.[11] Consider trading your pasta for this creamy porridge more often—and be sure to enjoy it with olive oil or a few shavings of cheese. The body only absorbs beta-carotene when it's eaten with a little bit of fat.

TOMATO-BRAISED CHICKEN THIGHS WITH CAPERS

This dish provides enough sauce to serve with polenta or a serving of whole grain pasta of your choice.

PREP TIME: 10 MINUTES / TOTAL TIME: 55 MINUTES / SERVES 4

1	tablespoon olive oil
8	boneless, skinless chicken thighs, trimmed
¼	teaspoon kosher salt
¼	teaspoon ground black pepper
1	onion, sliced
4	tablespoons drained capers, divided
1	clove garlic, minced
½	cup dry red wine or chicken broth
1	can (28 ounces) diced tomatoes
1	sprig fresh oregano or 1 teaspoon dried
2	tablespoons sliced fresh basil

1. In a Dutch oven or large wide-bottom pot over medium-high heat, warm the oil. Season the chicken with the salt and pepper. Add it to the pot, in batches, and cook until browned on both sides and it releases easily from the pot, 8 to 10 minutes total. Remove to a plate.

2. Reduce the heat to medium. Add the onion, 3 tablespoons of the capers, and the garlic. Cook, stirring frequently, until the onion is tender, 2 to 3 minutes.

3. Add the wine or broth and scrape up the browned bits from the bottom of the pot. Cook until the liquid is nearly cooked away, 4 to 5 minutes. Add the tomatoes and oregano and bring to a simmer.

4. Nestle the chicken into the tomato mixture and add the collected juices from the plate. Reduce the heat to maintain a bare simmer, cover, and cook until the chicken reaches 165°F in the thickest portion, about 15 minutes. Chop the remaining 1 tablespoon capers and sprinkle with the basil over the chicken before serving.

Per serving: 352 calories, 40 g protein, 14 g carbohydrates, 7 g sugars, 12 g total fat, 2.5 g saturated fat, 3 g fiber, 979 mg sodium

NOTE: This recipe is customizable to serve however many people you have to feed. Count on 2 chicken thighs per person. The amount of sauce in this recipe can braise up to 12 thighs. If you are cooking for a crowd, transfer the heated tomato mixture from Step 3 to a large baking dish or roasting pan and bake the chicken, covered, in a 375°F oven for 15 to 20 minutes.

OUZO MUSSELS

These delicious mussels are even more delicious when served with crusty bread to soak up all the flavorful broth.

PREP TIME: 10 MINUTES / TOTAL TIME: 25 MINUTES / SERVES 4

1 tablespoon olive oil
2 shallots, chopped
4 cloves garlic, sliced
1 pound mussels, scrubbed and debearded (see note on page 103)
1 cup low-sodium chicken broth or water
½ cup ouzo
 Grated peel of 1 lemon
2 tablespoons chopped fresh flat-leaf parsley

1. In a large pot over medium heat, warm the oil. Cook the shallots and garlic until softened, 5 minutes. Increase the heat and add the mussels, broth or water, and ouzo. Cover, bring to a boil, and cook until the mussels have opened, about 8 minutes.

2. Discard any unopened mussels. Sprinkle the lemon peel and parsley over the top. Serve the mussels with their broth.

Per serving: 238 calories, 16 g protein, 22 g carbohydrates, 10 g sugars, 6 g total fat, 1 g saturated fat, 0 g fiber, 344 mg sodium

235

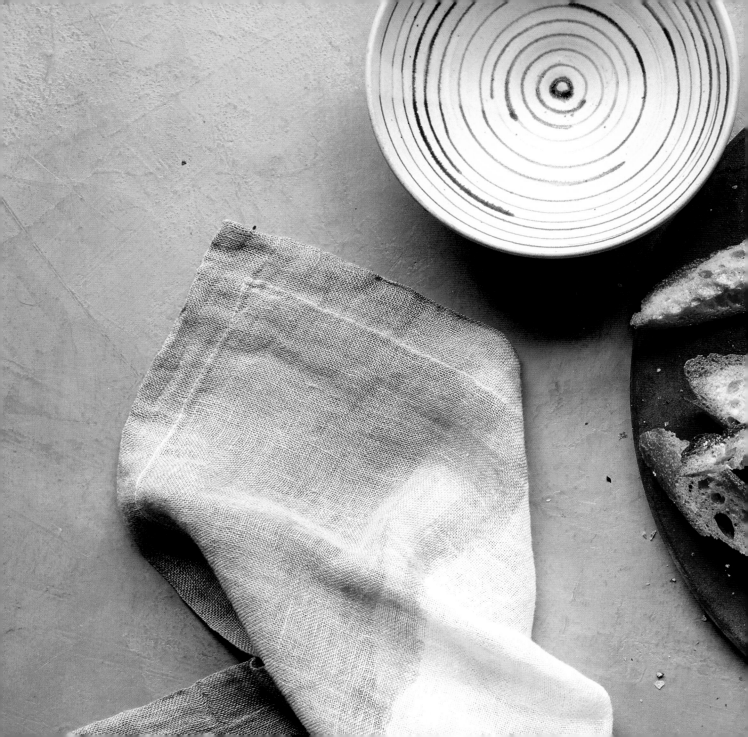

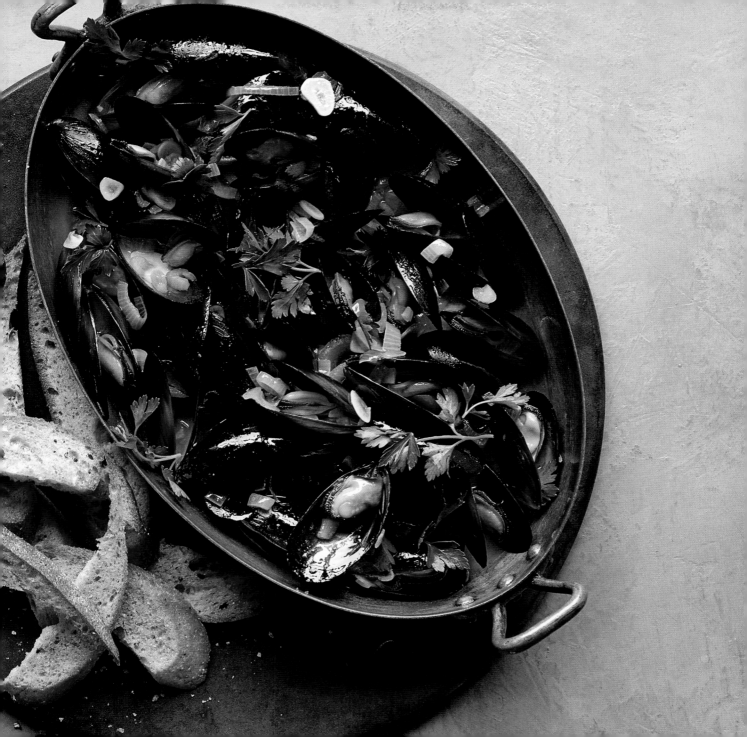

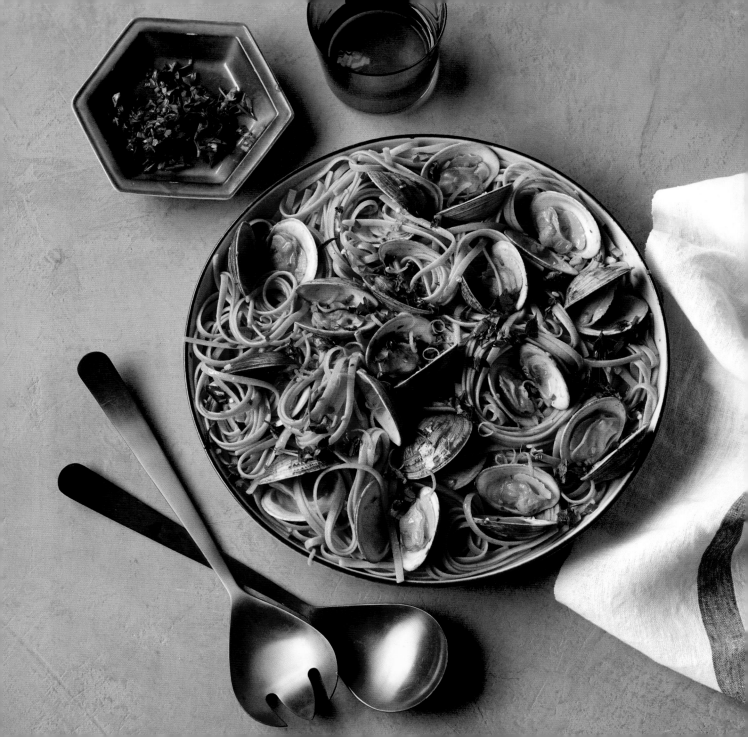

LINGUINE WITH CLAMS

Briny fresh clams meet a garlicky wine sauce in this traditional linguine con le vongole. The clam extract, or liquor as it's called, helps to flavor the sauce and, in turn, the linguine.

PREP TIME: 10 MINUTES / TOTAL TIME: 25 MINUTES / SERVES 6

1 pound whole wheat linguine
2 tablespoons olive oil
3 cloves garlic, minced
¼ teaspoon red-pepper flakes
½ cup dry white wine
1 tablespoon lemon juice
4 dozen littleneck clams, scrubbed
¼ cup chopped fresh flat-leaf parsley
2 teaspoons grated lemon peel (optional)

1. Cook the linguine to 1 minute under al dente according to package directions.

2. Meanwhile, in a large skillet over medium heat, warm the oil. Add the garlic and pepper flakes and cook until fragrant, about 1 minute.

3. Add the wine, lemon juice, and clams. Cover and cook, shaking the skillet occasionally, until all the clams have opened, 6 to 7 minutes. (Discard any that do not open.)

4. When the pasta is done, drain it and reserve ½ cup of the cooking water. Add the pasta to the skillet, tossing the pasta to coat in the sauce. Add the reserved cooking water if the pasta seems dry. Sprinkle with the parsley and lemon peel, if using.

Per serving: 384 calories, 22 g protein, 60 g carbohydrates, 3 g sugars, 6 g total fat, 1 g saturated fat, 9 g fiber, 440 mg sodium

239

NOTE: If you'd rather not deal with clamshells, swap the fresh clams for two 10-ounce cans of whole baby clams and use them, juice and all, in Step 3.

SHRIMP SAGANAKI

This dish is named after the cooking vessel it is made in: A Greek saganaki is a small double-handled frying pan or skillet.

PREP TIME: 10 MINUTES / TOTAL TIME: 30 MINUTES / SERVES 4

2   tablespoons extra-virgin olive oil
2   shallots, thinly sliced
6   plum tomatoes, coarsely chopped
    Pinch of kosher salt
    Pinch of ground black pepper
¼   cup ouzo
1½ pounds shrimp, peeled and deveined
2   tablespoons chopped fresh flat-leaf parsley
1   tablespoon chopped fresh dill
4   Whole Wheat Pitas (page 164), toasted

1. In a medium heavy-bottom skillet over medium heat, warm the oil. Cook the shallots until translucent, about 5 minutes. Add the tomatoes, salt, and pepper and cook, stirring, until the pot is mostly dry, about 5 minutes.
2. Stir in the ouzo and cook until reduced by half, about 2 minutes. Space the shrimp around the skillet, cover, and cook until the shrimp are opaque, about 5 minutes.
3. Toss in the parsley and dill and serve with the pita.

Per serving: 435 calories, 32 g protein, 52 g carbohydrates, 7 g sugars, 11 g total fat, 2 g saturated fat, 5 g fiber, 1,456 mg sodium

240

CHICKEN AND OLIVES WITH COUSCOUS

It might seem unusual to add olives before the dish is cooked. But the results are truly delicious: Their rich, briny flavor is infused into the chicken and couscous.

PREP TIME: 15 MINUTES / TOTAL TIME: 1 HOUR 15 MINUTES / SERVES 6

2   tablespoons olive oil, divided
8   bone-in, skin-on chicken thighs
½   teaspoon kosher salt
¼   teaspoon ground black pepper
2   cloves garlic, chopped
1   small red onion, chopped
1   red bell pepper, seeded and chopped
1   green bell pepper, seeded and chopped
1   tablespoon fresh thyme leaves
2   teaspoons fresh oregano leaves
1   can (28 ounces) no-salt-added diced tomatoes
1   cup low-sodium chicken broth
1   cup pitted green olives, coarsely chopped
2   cups whole wheat couscous
    Chopped flat-leaf parsley, for garnish

1. Preheat the oven to 350°F.

2. In a large ovenproof or cast-iron skillet over medium heat, warm 1 tablespoon of the oil. Pat the chicken thighs dry with a paper towel, season with the salt and black pepper, and cook, turning once, until golden and crisp, 8 to 10 minutes per side. Remove the chicken from the skillet and set aside.

3. Add the remaining 1 tablespoon oil to the skillet. Cook the garlic, onion, bell peppers, thyme, and oregano until softened, about 5 minutes. Add the tomatoes and broth and bring to a boil. Return the chicken to the skillet, add the olives, cover, and place the skillet in the oven. Roast until the chicken is tender and a thermometer inserted in the thickest part registers 165°F, 40 to 50 minutes.

4. While the chicken is cooking, prepare the couscous according to package directions.

5. To serve, pile the couscous on a serving platter and nestle the chicken on top. Pour the vegetables and any pan juices over the chicken and couscous. Sprinkle with the parsley and serve.

Per serving: 481 calories, 29 g protein, 61 g carbohydrates, 7 g sugars, 15 g total fat, 2.5 g saturated fat, 11 g fiber, 893 mg sodium

241

CHORIZO, SHRIMP, AND CHICKPEA STEW

It's common to enjoy cured meats like chorizo in Spain, but the portions are always modest. This flavorful stew only has about an ounce of chorizo per serving.

PREP TIME: 10 MINUTES / TOTAL TIME: 55 MINUTES / SERVES 6

¼ cup extra-virgin olive oil
1 large white onion, diced
4 cloves garlic, minced
6 ounces Spanish chorizo, casings removed and sliced
2 teaspoons sweet or hot smoked paprika, plus more to taste
Pinch of kosher salt
2 bay leaves
2 sprigs fresh thyme
½ teaspoon dried oregano
4 cups low-sodium chicken broth
1 can (14.5 ounces) no-salt-added diced tomatoes
2 cans (15 ounces each) no-salt-added chickpeas, drained and rinsed (see note on page 80)
1 pound curly kale, stems removed and coarsely chopped
1 pound shrimp, peeled and deveined

1. In a large saucepan over medium-low heat, warm the oil until shimmering. Cook the onion and garlic until the onion is golden brown, about 15 minutes. Add the chorizo, paprika, and salt and cook until the flavors have melded, about 5 minutes. Stir in the bay leaves, thyme, and oregano and cook until fragrant, 2 minutes.

2. Add the broth and tomatoes and bring to a boil. Reduce the heat to a simmer and add the chickpeas and kale and cook until the kale is tender, about 10 minutes. Stir in the shrimp and simmer until they turn pink and opaque, about 4 minutes.

3. Remove and discard the bay leaves and the thyme sprigs. Season to taste with more paprika and ladle into bowls.

Per serving: 371 calories, 26 g protein, 31 g carbohydrates, 4 g sugars, 17 g total fat, 3 g saturated fat, 6 g fiber, 891 mg sodium

BAKED RED SNAPPER WITH POTATOES AND TOMATOES

Don't fear the whole fish! Gorgeous red snapper can readily be found at fish markets and well-stocked supermarkets. Look for clear—not cloudy—eyes and bright red—not grey or purple—gills. It should already come cleaned and gutted, but ask the fishmonger to scale it and remove the fins for you.

PREP TIME: 10 MINUTES / TOTAL TIME: 1 HOUR / SERVES 4

5   sprigs fresh thyme, divided
2   sprigs fresh oregano, divided
1½ pounds new potatoes, halved (or quartered if large)
4   Roma tomatoes, quartered lengthwise
1   tablespoon plus 1 teaspoon olive oil
4   cloves garlic, halved, divided
1¼ teaspoons kosher salt, divided
¾   teaspoon ground black pepper, divided
1   cleaned whole red snapper (about 2 pounds), scaled and fins removed
½–1 lemon, sliced
4   cups (4 ounces) baby spinach

1. Preheat the oven to 350°F.

2. Strip the leaves off 2 sprigs thyme and 1 sprig oregano and chop. In a 9" x 13" baking dish, toss the potatoes and tomatoes with 1 tablespoon of the oil, the chopped thyme and oregano leaves, 2 cloves of the garlic, 1 teaspoon of the salt, and ½ teaspoon of the pepper.

3. Cut 3 or 4 diagonal slashes in the skin on both sides of the snapper. Rub the skin with the remaining 1 teaspoon oil. Sprinkle the cavity of the snapper with the remaining ¼ teaspoon salt and pepper. Fill it with the lemon slices, the remaining thyme and oregano sprigs, and the remaining 2 cloves garlic. Sprinkle the outside of the snapper with a pinch of salt and pepper. Set the fish on the vegetables.

4. Cover the baking dish with foil and bake for 20 minutes. Remove the foil and continue baking until the potatoes are tender and the fish flakes easily with a fork, 20 to 25 minutes.

5. Transfer the fish to a serving platter. Toss the spinach with the tomatoes and potatoes in the baking dish, until wilted.

6. Using forks, peel the skin off the fish fillets. Scatter the vegetables around the fish and serve.

Per serving: 345 calories, 39 g protein, 33 g carbohydrates, 4 g sugars, 6 g total fat, 1 g saturated fat, 5 g fiber, 782 mg sodium

ROAST PORK LOIN WITH JUNIPER BERRIES AND HONEY

Juniper berries are common in an Italian pantry, adding a sharp flavor to dishes. You can find them with the spices in some grocery stores or substitute a bay leaf and a splash of gin.

PREP TIME: 5 MINUTES / TOTAL TIME: 1 HOUR / SERVES 6

2   cloves garlic, chopped
3   or 4 leaves fresh sage, chopped
1   tablespoon chopped fresh rosemary
1   tablespoon juniper berries, crushed
2   tablespoons olive oil, divided
1   bone-in pork loin roast (3–4 pounds), trimmed
1   cup low-sodium chicken broth
2   teaspoons honey
½   teaspoon kosher salt
¼   teaspoon ground black pepper

1. Preheat the oven to 400°F.

2. In a small bowl, stir together the garlic, sage, rosemary, juniper berries, and 1 table-spoon of the oil. Rub this mixture all over the pork loin and place in a large baking dish.

3. Roast the pork loin, turning the meat over once, until a thermometer placed in the center reads 150°F, about 50 minutes. Remove the pork from the baking dish and set aside to rest.

4. Strain the juices from the baking dish into a small saucepan. Add the broth, honey, salt, and pepper and bring to a boil. Reduce the heat to a simmer and cook until thickened, about 8 minutes.

5. To serve, slice the pork and drizzle the sauce over top.

Per serving: 366 calories, 50 g protein, 4 g carbohydrates, 2 g sugars, 16 g total fat, 4 g saturated fat, 0 g fiber, 342 mg sodium

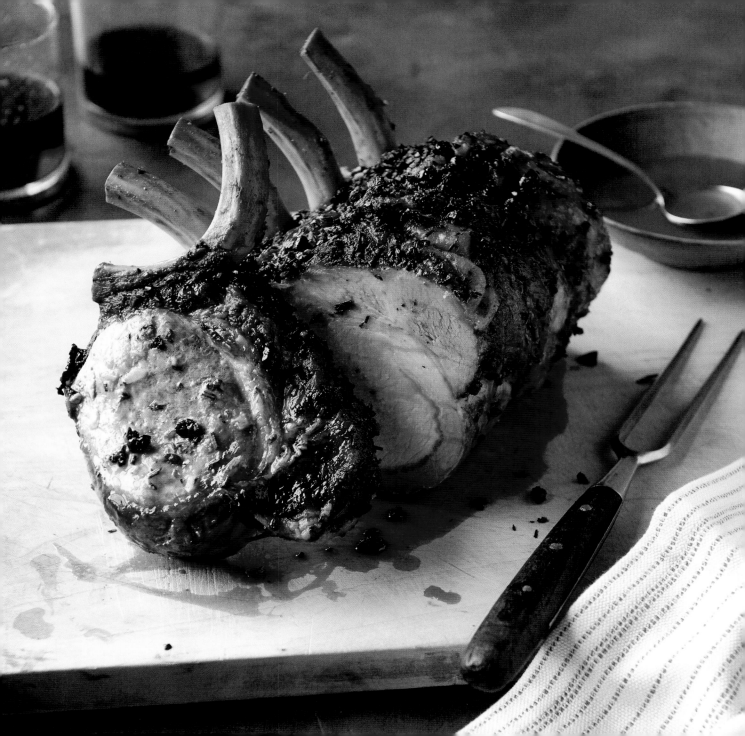

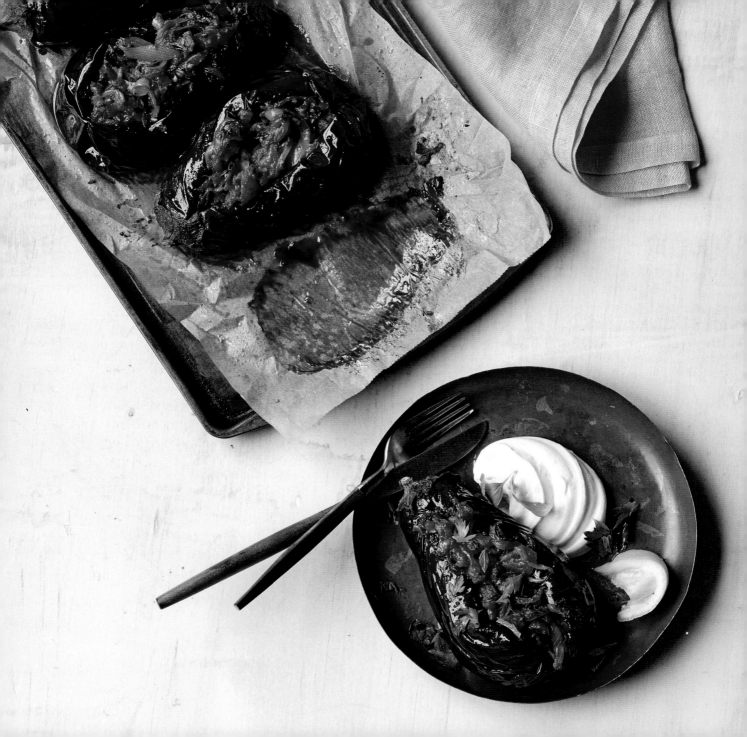

IMAM BAYILDI (STUFFED EGGPLANT WITH TOMATOES AND HERBS)

Legend has it that the priest fainted from the absolute deliciousness of this eggplant dish, and that's how it got its name, which translates to mean: "The Fainting Priest."

PREP TIME: 10 MINUTES / TOTAL TIME: 1 HOUR 15 MINUTES / SERVES 4

4 small eggplant
¼ cup extra-virgin olive oil, divided
1 large onion, thinly sliced
4 cloves garlic, minced
1 can (28 ounces) whole peeled plum tomatoes, drained and coarsely chopped
½ teaspoon ground cumin
¼ teaspoon ground cinnamon
Generous pinch of kosher salt
Generous pinch of ground black pepper
½ cup chopped fresh flat-leaf parsley
¼ cup chopped fresh basil
2 tablespoons chopped fresh mint
4 lemon wedges
½ cup low-fat Greek yogurt or labneh

1. Preheat the oven to 400°F. Lightly grease a large rimmed baking sheet with olive oil.

2. On one side of the eggplant, slice off a very thin piece of the flesh to make a flat surface so they don't roll around. Place the eggplant on the baking sheet. Make a lengthwise incision into the center of the eggplant, making sure not to cut all the way through. Roast until the skin begins to shrivel and the flesh is almost completely tender, about 25 minutes. Remove from the oven and carefully drain any excess liquid within the cavity.

3. Meanwhile, in a large skillet over medium heat, warm 2 tablespoons of the oil. Cook the onion and garlic until the onion is golden brown, about 10 minutes. Add the tomatoes, cumin, cinnamon, salt, and pepper and cook to meld the flavors, about 5 minutes. Remove the skillet from the heat and stir in the herbs.

4. Fill the eggplants with the tomato mixture, drizzle with the remaining 2 tablespoons oil, cover the baking sheet with foil, and cook until the eggplant is completely fork-tender, about 40 minutes. Serve with the lemon wedges and yogurt or labneh.

Per serving: 254 calories, 7 g protein, 26 g carbohydrates, 13 g sugars, 15 g total fat, 3 g saturated fat, 9 g fiber, 548 mg sodium

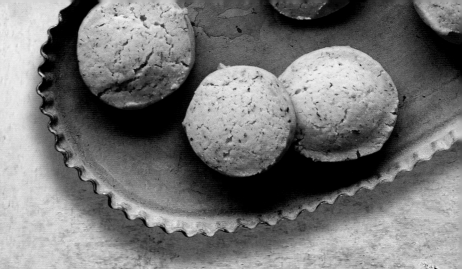

Chapter 8
Dessert

If you're looking for a tasty treat, good news: Many Mediterranean meals finish off with something sweet, and you'll find plenty of scrumptious options in this chapter. But the treats on most Mediterranean tables tend to look a little different than what you'll often find here at home. Here's what sets them apart and why it's worth making your desserts more Mediterranean.

• **EVERYDAY DESSERTS ARE SIMPLE.** Decadent cookies, cakes, and pastries certainly make an appearance for special occasions, but everyday desserts in the Mediterranean are often based around fresh fruit—think wine-poached pears, grilled stone fruit, macerated berries, or even simple sorbets, which don't need much added sugar to taste delicious.

• **CHEESE CAN BE DESSERT.** With so many delicious options to choose from, it's not uncommon for cheese to show up at the end of the meal. Often, it's paired with dried fruit or preserves, serving up a satisfying combo of sweet and salty flavors.

• **SO CAN FRESH FRUIT.** Keeping with the spirit of moderation, sometimes dessert is simply a cluster of juicy grapes, a bowl of jewel-like berries, or a fragrant clementine. And when you stick to offerings that are in season, the flavor is just as sweet and satisfying as a richer treat. Try it!

• **THE PORTIONS ARE SMALLER.** Think, a scoop of sorbet, a cube of cheese, or a tiny tea cookie. Keeping with the spirit of moderation, Mediterranean-style desserts are often just a few flavorful bites. Smaller helpings mean that you can feel good about enjoying dessert more often. Plus, you'll leave the table feeling comfortable and satisfied instead of overly full.

Recipes

CHERRY-ALMOND CLAFOUTIS

This classic French dessert tastes like a cross between cake and a creamy custard. Cherries are traditional, but feel free to experiment with other summer fruits—like blueberries or sliced plums.

PREP TIME: 5 MINUTES / TOTAL TIME: 90 MINUTES / SERVES 8

1 tablespoon unsalted butter, cut into small pieces
1 cup whole milk
⅔ cup unbleached all-purpose flour, sifted
¼ cup sugar, divided
¼ cup heavy cream
3 eggs
⅛ teaspoon pure almond extract
⅛ teaspoon table salt
3 cups fresh cherries, pitted
⅓ cup sliced almonds

1. Preheat the oven to 400°F. Grease a shallow round ceramic 11" gratin dish with a little butter.

2. In the bowl of an electric stand mixer fitted with a whisk attachment, add the milk, flour, 3 tablespoons of the sugar, the cream, eggs, almond extract, and salt and beat on medium speed to combine and aerate, about 5 minutes.

3. Arrange the cherries in the gratin dish and pour the batter over the top. Bake for 15 minutes.

4. Sprinkle the almonds all over the top, followed by the remaining 1 tablespoon sugar and the butter pieces. Bake until the clafoutis is puffed and golden brown around the edges, about 40 minutes. A toothpick inserted in the center will come out clean.

5. Transfer to a rack to cool for 20 minutes. Scoop out to serve.

Per serving: 205 calories, 6 g protein, 26 g carbohydrates, 15 g sugars, 9 g total fat, 4 g saturated fat, 2 g fiber, 79 mg sodium

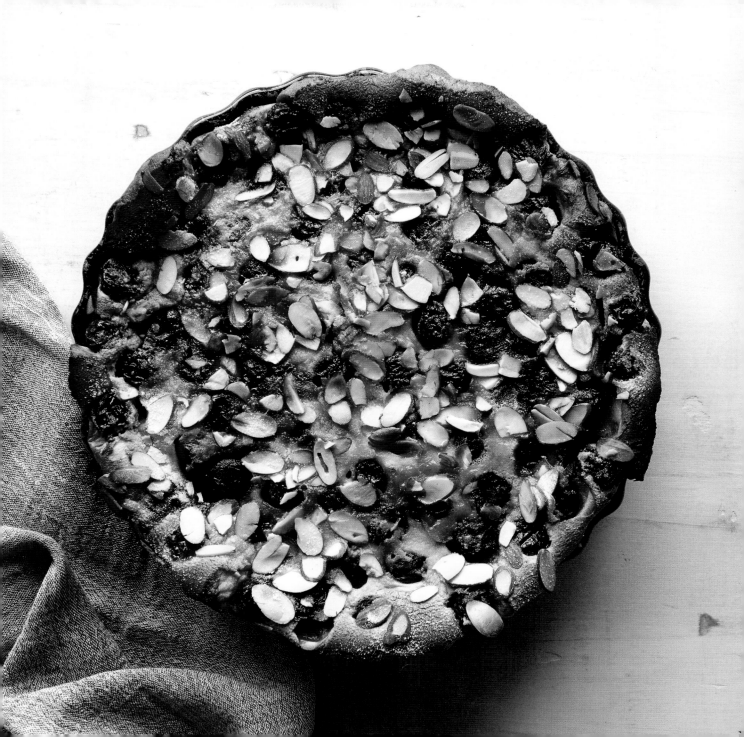

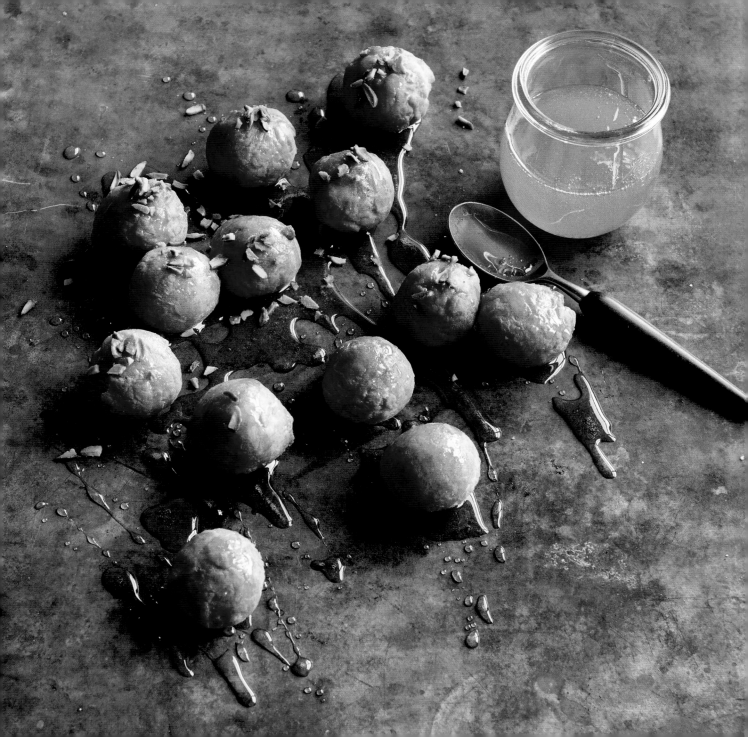

LOUKOUMADES
(HONEY DUMPLINGS)

These honey dumplings are particularly popular on Crete but can be found in Turkey, Greece, Cyprus, and Egypt. We've simplified the batter to skip the yeast and increased the nutrition with whole wheat flour. Keep in mind that they are still fried in oil, so keep your portions small.

PREP TIME: 10 MINUTES / TOTAL TIME: 45 MINUTES / SERVES 24 (2 PER SERVING)

4 cups olive oil or vegetable oil
I cup all-purpose flour
¾ cup whole wheat flour
½ cup sugar
I teaspoon baking powder
½ teaspoon table salt
½ teaspoon ground cardamom
¼ teaspoon baking soda
⅓ cup buttermilk
⅓ cup fresh orange juice
I egg
2 tablespoons olive oil
½ cup honey
3 tablespoons fresh lemon juice
I teaspoon ground cinnamon
2 tablespoons finely ground walnuts or pistachios, or sesame seeds

1. In a 4-quart heavy-bottom pot fitted with an oil thermometer over medium heat, warm the 4 cups oil until it reaches 375ºF. (This will take about 15 minutes.) Line a baking sheet with paper towels.

2. In a large bowl, whisk together the flours, sugar, baking powder, salt, cardamom, and baking soda.

3. In a separate medium bowl, whisk together the buttermilk, orange juice, egg, and the 2 tablespoons oil. Add the buttermilk mixture to the flour mixture and stir until just combined. The dough will be sticky.

4. Turn the dough out onto a well-floured work surface and with floured hands, pat down into a square ½" thick. With a floured pastry cutter, cut the dough into 1" squares.

(continued)

(continued from page 253)

5. With floured hands, gently roll 8 of the dough squares into balls and carefully lower them into the oil. Fry until deeply golden, about 50 seconds on each side. (They should turn over all on their own.) Constantly monitor the heat to maintain oil temperature.

6. Remove the dumplings with a slotted spoon to the baking sheet to drain. Repeat with the remaining dough.

7. Meanwhile, in a small saucepan over medium heat, warm the honey, lemon juice, and cinnamon, stirring until combined, about 5 minutes.

8. Transfer the dumplings to a serving platter and drizzle with the warm honey mixture. Top with the nuts or sesame seeds. Alternatively, serve 2 loukoumades per person, drizzled with 1 teaspoon of the honey syrup and a pinch of nuts or sesame seeds.

Per serving: 170 calories, 2 g protein, 18 g carbohydrates, 11 g sugars, 11 g total fat, 1.5 g saturated fat, 1 g fiber, 90 mg sodium

254

HONEY

Nature's original sweetener might also be one of the best for you. In addition to serving up trace minerals like magnesium and calcium, honey is rich in polyphenols that could play a role in lowering blood pressure and improving cholesterol.[1] The sticky stuff is also teeming with antibacterial agents, as well as probiotic bacteria that recent Japanese research found could help stimulate the immune system.[2] *And* it serves up *pre*biotics, a type of sugar that feeds probiotics and appears to play a role in suppressing stress hormones.[3] Eating local honey even exposes you to tiny amounts of local pollen, which some experts suspect could make you less sensitive to seasonal allergens. More research is needed to determine whether honey's pollen is actually potent enough to ease springtime sniffles, but enjoying it during allergy season certainly won't hurt! For the biggest benefits, seek out locally produced raw, unfiltered honey: Most commercial products are filtered and pasteurized, which significantly slashes honey's nutritional potential.[4] And remember: Like all sweets, honey is best enjoyed in moderation!

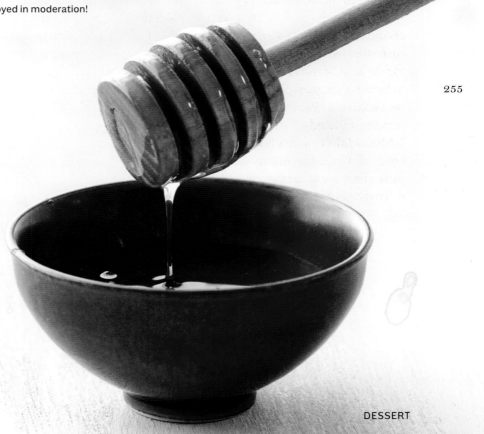

ROSEMARY-ORANGE OLIVE OIL CAKE

This cake is the perfect end to a special-occasion meal—it's flavorful and beautiful. For a different flavor, replace the rosemary with 1 tablespoon dried lavender and replace the oranges with lemons.

PREP TIME: 10 MINUTES / TOTAL TIME: 1 HOUR / SERVES 12

2 oranges
1½ cups all-purpose flour
1 cup sugar
1 teaspoon kosher salt
½ teaspoon baking soda
½ teaspoon baking powder
¾ cup extra-virgin olive oil
¾ cup fat-free milk
3 eggs
1 teaspoon chopped fresh rosemary
1 tablespoon chopped roasted unsalted pistachios

1. Preheat the oven to 350°F. Coat a 9" cake pan with cooking spray and line the bottom with parchment paper. Grate the peel of 1 orange, juice, and set aside. Cut the peel from the other orange, slice the fruit into ¼" thick rounds, and set aside.

2. In a medium bowl, whisk the flour, sugar, salt, baking soda, and baking powder. In a large bowl, whisk the orange juice, grated orange peel, oil, milk, eggs, and rosemary. Add the dry ingredients and whisk until just combined.

3. Pour the batter into the pan and bake until the top is golden and a cake tester inserted in the middle comes out clean, 40 to 45 minutes. Remove the cake from the oven and transfer to a rack to cool for 10 minutes. Run a knife around the edge of the pan, invert the cake onto the rack, and invert one more time onto a serving plate. Arrange the orange slices on top, sprinkle with the pistachios, and let cool completely.

Per serving: 285 calories, 4 g protein, 32 g carbohydrates, 20 g sugars, 16 g total fat, 2.5 g saturated fat, 1 g fiber, 258 mg sodium

256

ORANGES

Oranges are a skin superfood! A medium orange serves up more than a day's worth of vitamin C, which the body uses to make the skin-firming protein collagen and to fight the skin-damaging effects of environmental stressors like pollution and the sun's UV rays.[5] The fiber from the orange flesh helps fill you up longer and stave off blood sugar spikes.

TAHINI BAKLAVA CUPS

Try out this flavorful update of the traditional baklava with the addition of creamy tahini—a sesame seed paste. To thaw phyllo cups, let sit at room temperature for 2 hours or in the refrigerator overnight.

PREP TIME: 10 MINUTES / TOTAL TIME: 35 MINUTES / SERVES 8 (2 PER SERVING)

1   box (about 16) mini phyllo dough cups, thawed
⅓   cup tahini
¼   cup shelled pistachios or walnuts, chopped, plus more for garnish
4   tablespoons honey, divided
1   teaspoon ground cinnamon
    Pinch of kosher salt
½   teaspoon rosewater (optional)

1. Preheat the oven to 350°F. Remove the phyllo cups from the packaging and place on a large rimmed baking sheet.

2. In a small bowl, stir together the tahini, nuts, 1 tablespoon of the honey, the cinnamon, and salt. Divide this mixture among the phyllo cups and top each with a few more nuts. Bake until golden and warmed through, 10 minutes. Remove from the oven and cool for 5 minutes.

3. Meanwhile, in a small saucepan or in a microwaveable bowl, stir together the remaining 3 tablespoons honey and the rosewater, if using, and heat until warmed, about 5 minutes over medium heat on the stove top or 30 seconds on high in the microwave. Arrange the phyllo cups on a serving platter and drizzle the warmed honey over the top. Serve warm or at room temperature.

Per serving: 176 calories, 4 g protein, 17 g carbohydrates, 9 g sugars, 11 g total fat, 1.5 g saturated fat, 1 g fiber, 38 mg sodium

FRUIT, NUT, AND CHEESE PLATTERS

Composed of several different items and designed for guests to "choose their own adventure," a cheese platter is made of several different items and ends the meal on a flavorful and sophisticated note. Platters can have any or all the following categories!

FRESH FRUITS (½ CUP PER SERVING)

Grapes: 52 calories, 1 g protein, 14 g carbohydrates, 12 g sugars, 0 g total fat, 0 g saturated fat, 1 g fiber, 2 mg sodium

Melon: 27 calories, 1 g protein, 7 g carbohydrates, 6 g sugars, 0 g total fat, 0 g saturated fat, 1 g fiber, 13 mg sodium

Berries: 32 calories, 1 g protein, 7 g carbohydrates, 3 g sugars, 0 g total fat, 0 g saturated fat, 4 g fiber, 1 mg sodium

Apples: 47 calories, 0 g protein, 13 g carbohydrates, 10 g sugars, 0 g total fat, 0 g saturated fat, 2 g fiber, 1 mg sodium

Pears: 51 calories, 0 g protein, 14 g carbohydrates, 9 g sugars, 0 g total fat, 0 g saturated fat, 3 g fiber, 1 mg sodium

Figs: 59 calories, 1 g protein, 15 g carbohydrates, 13 g sugars, 0 g total fat, 0 g saturated fat, 2 g fiber, 1 mg sodium

CHEESES (1 OUNCE PER SERVING)

Manchego: 129 calories, 7 g protein, 0 g carbohydrates, 0 g sugars, 11 g total fat, 7 g saturated fat, 0 g fiber, 242 mg sodium

Goat cheese: 103 calories, 6 g protein, 0 g carbohydrates, 0 g sugars, 9 g total fat, 6 g saturated fat, 0 g fiber, 146 mg sodium

Feta: 75 calories, 4 g protein, 1 g carbohydrates, 1 g sugars, 6 g total fat, 4 g saturated fat, 0 g fiber, 316 mg sodium

Gouda: 101 calories, 7 g protein, 0 g carbohydrates, 1 g sugars, 8 g total fat, 5 g saturated fat, 0 g fiber, 232 mg sodium

Parmigiano-Reggiano: 12 calories, 11 g protein, 1 g carbohydrates, 0 g sugars, 8 g total fat, 5 g saturated fat, 0 g fiber, 428 mg sodium

NUTS (1 OUNCE PER SERVING)

Almonds: 163 calories, 6 g protein, 6 g carbohydrates, 1 g sugars, 15 g total fat, 1 g saturated fat, 4 g fiber, 0 mg sodium

Marcona almonds: 185 calories, 6 g protein, 5 g carbohydrates, 2 g sugars, 17 g total fat, 1 g saturated fat, 3 g fiber, 111 mg sodium

Walnuts: 185 calories, 4 g protein, 4 g carbohydrates, 1 g sugars, 19 g total fat, 2 g saturated fat, 2 g fiber, 1 mg sodium

Pistachios: 161 calories, 6 g protein, 8 g carbohydrates, 2 g sugars, 13 g total fat, 2 g saturated fat, 3 g fiber, 2 mg sodium

Hazelnuts: 178 calories, 4 g protein, 5 g carbohydrates, 1 g sugars, 17 g total fat, 1 g saturated fat, 3 g fiber, 0 mg sodium

SWEETS (1 TABLESPOON PER SERVING)

Jams: 50 calories, 0 g protein, 13 g carbohydrates, 12 g sugars, 0 g total fat, 0 g saturated fat, 0 g fiber, 0 mg sodium

Jellies: 50 calories, 0 g protein, 13 g carbohydrates, 12 g sugars, 0 g total fat, 0 g saturated fat, 0 g fiber, 0 mg sodium

Compotes: 34 calories, 0 g protein, 9 g carbohydrates, 7 g sugars, 0 g total fat, 0 g saturated fat, 1 g fiber, 1 mg sodium

Pastes, such as the Quince Paste on page 261

CRACKERS (1 OUNCE PER SERVING)

Toasted pitas: 130 calories, 3 g protein, 19 g carbohydrates, 1 g sugars, 4 g total fat, 0 g saturated fat, 1 g fiber, 242 mg sodium

Water crackers: 117 calories, 3 g protein, 22 g carbohydrates, 0 g sugars, 3 g total fat, 1 g saturated fat, 1 g fiber, 167 mg sodium

Crispbreads: 115 calories, 3 g protein, 24 g carbohydrates, 1 g sugars, 0 g total fat, 0 g saturated fat, 1 g fiber, 1 mg sodium

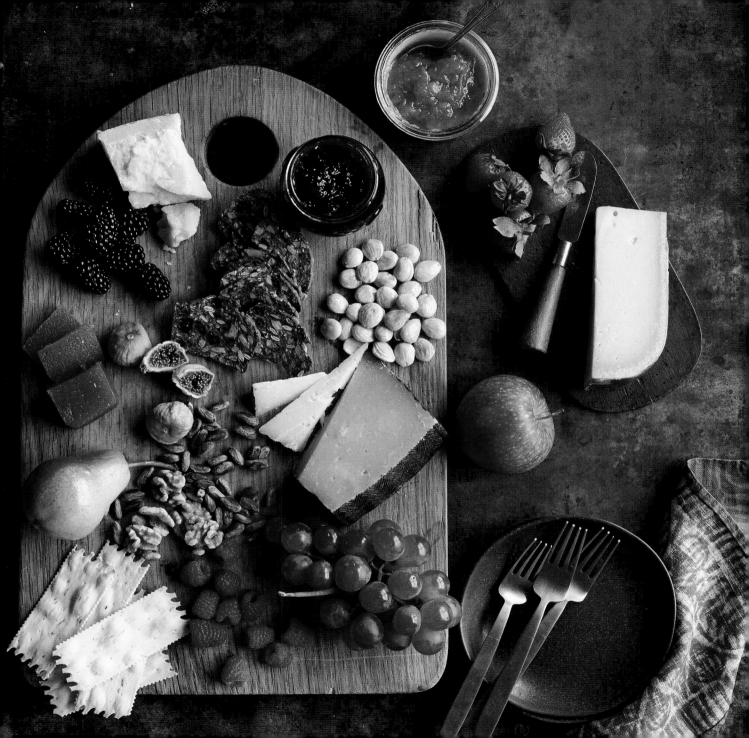

NUTS

Rich, crunchy, and satisfying, nuts just might be nature's perfect snack. People who nosh on nuts daily live longer than those who skip out, according to Harvard research.[6] Perhaps because higher nut consumption fights inflammation and insulin resistance and is linked to everything from a lower risk of heart disease to type 2 diabetes to colon cancer.

And forget those fears about nuts making you gain weight. Thanks to their combination of protein, fiber, and healthy fat, it only takes a handful to fill you up and keep you satisfied for hours. Findings show that regular nut eaters tend to weigh less,[7] and some research even suggests that nuts can help melt fat—especially the harmful kind around your belly.[8]

Walnuts, which are a staple in many Mediterranean dishes, might be particularly beneficial. Like fish, they're rich in omega-3 fatty acids, and they've been shown to lower levels of bad cholesterol by as much as 16 percent.[9] Still, variety is the spice of life, so make an effort to switch it up! From almonds to pistachios to walnuts, all nuts pack a tasty health punch. For the biggest benefits, pick plain, unsalted ones—salted or flavored varieties tend to be higher in sodium and sugar. Instead, season them yourself with a pinch of sea salt, herbs or spices, grated citrus peel, or even a drizzle of honey, if you'd like. The results will be better for you—not to mention even more delicious.

260

QUINCE PASTE

Quince, an applelike fruit, cannot be eaten raw. But when cooked, it has a delicious floral apple-pear flavor and its color deepens to a rosy pink. Quince paste is often eaten atop a slice of Manchego or other salty hard cheese as part of a dessert platter.

PREP TIME: 5 MINUTES / TOTAL TIME: 5 HOURS / SERVES 32 (A 2" X I" SLICE PER SERVING)

2 pounds quinces, peeled, cored, and coarsely chopped
½ vanilla bean, split and seeds scraped out
2 strips (2" each) lemon peel
2 cups sugar (more or less as needed)
2 tablespoons fresh lemon juice

1. In a large saucepan, add the quinces, vanilla bean pod and seeds, and lemon peel, cover with water, and bring to a boil. Reduce the heat to a simmer, cover, and cook until tender, about 40 minutes.

2. Drain the quinces in a colander, transfer with the lemon peel to a food processor, and discard the vanilla bean. Puree the fruit and lemon peel. Measure the puree by volume, return it to the saucepan, and add an equal volume of sugar. (For example, if you have 2 cups of puree, add 2 cups of sugar.)

3. Cook over low heat, stirring with a wooden spoon until the sugar has dissolved, about 5 minutes. Add the lemon juice and cook, stirring occasionally, until the puree becomes a very thick paste, about 2 hours.

4. Preheat the oven to 175°F. If your oven doesn't go this low, use the lowest temperature possible and expect a shorter cooking time. Line an 8" x 8" glass or ceramic baking dish with parchment and grease with olive oil.

5. Pour the quince paste into the dish and smooth the top with the wooden spoon. Bake until slightly dried and firm enough to slice, about 2 hours.

6. Remove from the oven and let cool to room temperature. Invert onto a cutting board and cut the quince paste into four 2"-wide strips. Wrap each strip in plastic wrap and refrigerate. Store in an airtight container for up to a month.

Per serving: 66 calories, 0 g protein, 17 g carbohydrates, 13 g sugars, 0 g total fat, 0 g saturated fat, 1 g fiber, 1 mg sodium

SPICE-POACHED PEARS

Poaching is the simplest means of transforming a fresh fruit into a spectacularly fancy dessert. Nobody needs to know you put everything in a pot and walked away! The fruit absorbs the flavors that have been infused into the poaching liquid. Though we call for red wine here, white wine works just as well—as would water.

PREP TIME: 10 MINUTES / TOTAL TIME: 1 HOUR 15 MINUTES / SERVES 6

6   Bosc pears, peeled
6   cups water
2   cups red wine
½   cup sugar
8   slices fresh ginger, ⅛" thick
½   vanilla bean, split and seeds scraped out
2   strips orange peel
1   cinnamon stick
2   star anise
2   cardamom pods
8   whole cloves
6   tablespoons chopped dried fruit, such as apricots, dates, figs, or crystallized ginger (optional)

1. If necessary for the pears to stand on end, trim a bit off their bottoms.

2. In a large (5-quart) pot that will have enough space to cover the pears completely with liquid without them touching each other, combine the water, wine, sugar, ginger, vanilla bean seeds and pod, orange peel, cinnamon stick, star anise, cardamom pods, and cloves. Bring to a simmer over medium-high heat, stirring until the sugar dissolves.

3. Reduce the heat to medium-low and add the pears. If there's not enough liquid, add another cup of water. If the pears float out of the liquid, cover them with a heavy plate to keep them submerged.

NOTES: To serve a larger crowd, or if you're looking for a smaller dessert after a heavy meal, halve the pears vertically, use a melon baller to scoop out the core, and poach as above. Serve ½ pear per person. A lovely accompaniment to this dessert is the whipped cream from the Espresso Granita with Whipped Cream on page 269.

262

PEARS

Pears don't just make for a light dessert, satisfying snack, or sweet addition to your salad. They're one of the best fruits for weight loss. When Harvard researchers tracked the eating habits and weight changes of some 133,000 adults for more than 2 decades, they found that frequent consumption of pears (and apples) was tied to greater weight loss than consumption of other fruits.[10] That could be because pears are some of the most fiber-rich fruits out there, serving up 6 grams per medium fruit. They also have a lower glycemic index than most other fruits—so they have a milder impact on blood sugar.

4. Cover the pot and simmer, turning the pears occasionally, until a spoon slides easily into the thickest portion, about 30 minutes. At this point, you can let the mixture cool and transfer the entire pot to the refrigerator to chill overnight before proceeding with Step 5. Otherwise, proceed with Step 5.

5. Remove the pears to a dish and cover with foil.

6. Strain the spices from the liquid. Return 3 cups liquid to the pot over medium-high heat. Boil until the syrup is reduced to $\frac{1}{2}$ cup, about 30 minutes.

7. Transfer the pears, standing up, to individual bowls. Spoon 4 teaspoons of the syrup over each pear, and sprinkle with 1 tablespoon dried fruit, if using.

Per serving: 151 calories, 1 g protein, 34 g carbohydrates, 24 g sugars, 0 g total fat, 0 g saturated fat, 6 g fiber, 5 mg sodium

263

GRILLED APRICOTS AND PLUMS WITH BASIL-HONEY YOGURT

Luscious, velvety apricots will maintain their firm texture even when warmed over the grill to create this quick and deceptively elegant light dessert.

½ cup low-fat plain Greek yogurt
2 tablespoons honey
2 tablespoons chopped fresh basil leaves
2 fresh apricots, halved
2 fresh plums, halved
1 tablespoon olive oil
Fresh mint leaves, for garnish (optional)

1. Coat a grill rack or grill pan with olive oil and prepare the grill to medium heat.

2. In a small bowl, stir together the yogurt, honey, and basil and set aside.

3. Brush the cut sides of the fruit with the oil. Grill the fruit, cut side down, until charred and collapsing, 5 to 8 minutes (the apricots will be done before the plums since they are smaller). Turn the fruit over and grill the other side for 3 to 4 minutes. Divide the fruit between 4 bowls and top with the basil-honey yogurt. Garnish with the mint leaves, if using.

Per serving: 104 calories, 3 g protein, 16 g carbohydrates, 15 g sugars, 4 g total fat, 1 g saturated fat, 1 g fiber, 10 mg sodium

264

PEAR AND CARDAMOM SORBET

Sorbets are traditionally served as palate cleansers during multicourse meals, but this decadent treat deserves center stage as a dessert. And you can make it without an ice cream maker!

PREP TIME: 5 MINUTES / TOTAL TIME: 6 HOURS (INCLUDING FREEZING TIME) / SERVES 5

2   large ripe pears, peeled, cored, and chopped
1½   cups water
½   cup sugar
1   tablespoon lemon juice
    Pinch of kosher salt
½   cup moscato, white wine, or water
½   teaspoon ground cardamom

1. In a 4-quart saucepan over medium-high heat, bring the pears, water, sugar, lemon juice, and salt to a simmer. Reduce the heat to a bare simmer (a few bubbles coming up to the surface), cover, and cook until the pears are very soft, about 35 minutes.

2. Transfer the mixture to a blender along with the wine or water and cardamom. Puree until smooth. Cool completely in the refrigerator, about 30 minutes.

3. *To process without an ice cream maker:* Transfer the sorbet to a 9" x 13" baking dish. Freeze until set, 3½ to 4 hours. Break the frozen puree into pieces and blend in a food processor until smooth. Return to the dish, spread out, and freeze for 1 hour more before serving. To store, transfer the sorbet to an airtight container and freeze until ready to use. Remove from the freezer a few minutes before eating. Store in the freezer for up to 3 months.

4. *To process with an ice cream maker:* Churn the sorbet in an ice cream maker according to the manufacturer's instructions. Transfer the sorbet to an airtight container and freeze until ready to use. Remove from the freezer a few minutes before eating. Store in the freezer for up to 3 months.

Per serving: 151 calories, 0 g protein, 36 g carbohydrates, 29 g sugars, 0 g total fat, 0 g saturated fat, 3 g fiber, 33 mg sodium

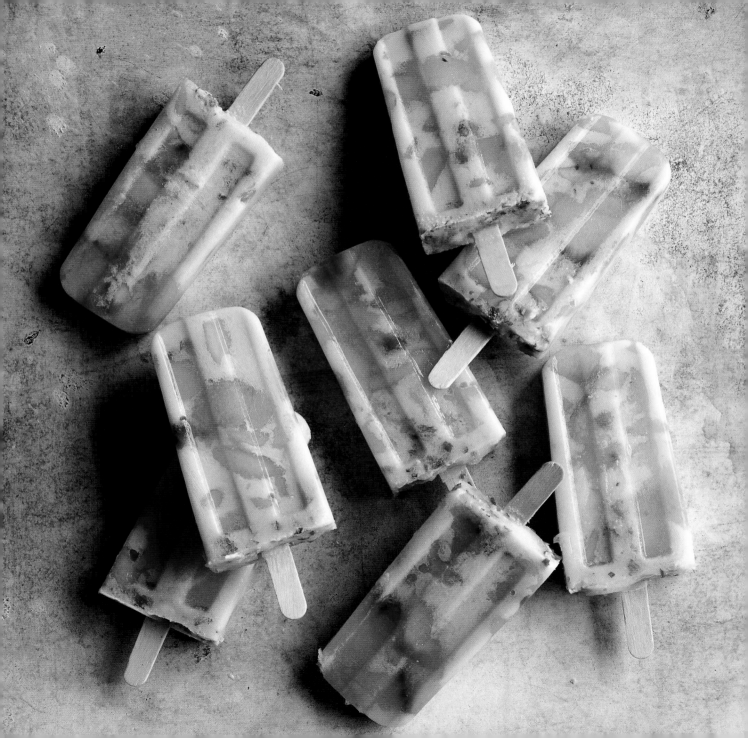

ALMOND-PEACH ICE POPS

These sweet and just a hint of tart pops are perfect for the kids on a hot summer night. If you don't have ice-pop molds, you can freeze these treats in small paper cups.

PREP TIME: 15 MINUTES / TOTAL TIME: 15 MINUTES PLUS FREEZING TIME / SERVES 10

1¾ cups unsweetened vanilla almond milk
2 teaspoons coconut oil, melted
1 tablespoon honey
4 or 5 ripe peaches, peeled and chopped
¼ cup roasted almonds, chopped

1. Whisk together the almond milk, oil, and honey.

2. Divide the peaches among the pop molds, ¼ to ⅓ cup per mold. Pour the almond milk mixture over the peaches to fill the mold. Insert sticks, sprinkle the tops with the almonds, and freeze overnight.

Per serving: 65 calories, 1 g protein, 9 g carbohydrates, 7 g sugars, 3 g total fat, 1 g saturated fat, 1 g fiber, 32 mg sodium

267

STRAWBERRY MASCARPONE PARFAITS

Summer strawberries taste even more delicious when they're marinated in almond and orange liqueur and layered with sweet mascarpone cream, toasted hazelnuts, and chocolate.

PREP TIME: 10 MINUTES / TOTAL TIME: 1 HOUR 30 MINUTES / SERVES 8

16 fresh strawberries, hulled and sliced
2   tablespoons amaretto, divided
1   tablespoon granulated sugar
2   teaspoons orange liqueur
¾   cup heavy cream
3   tablespoons confectioners' sugar
1   teaspoon grated orange peel
6   ounces mascarpone cheese
½   cup skinned hazelnuts, toasted and coarsely chopped
2   ounces dark chocolate, finely chopped

1. In a medium bowl, combine the strawberries, 1 tablespoon of the amaretto, the granulated sugar, and orange liqueur. Let the berries soak for about 1 hour but not more than 2 hours.

2. In a large bowl with an electric hand mixer, beat the cream with the confectioners' sugar until soft peaks form, about 4 minutes. Gently fold in the orange peel and the remaining 1 tablespoon amaretto.

3. In another large bowl, beat the mascarpone until softened, about 2 minutes. Fold the whipped cream into the mascarpone until completely combined.

4. In 8 small dessert glasses, layer the parfait in this order: mascarpone cream, a sprinkle of nuts and chocolate, and strawberry slices. Repeat until you reach the top of the glass, ending with cream sprinkled with nuts, chocolate, and a strawberry slice. Chill for at least 30 minutes before serving.

Per serving: 298 calories, 4 g protein, 16 g carbohydrates, 11 g sugars, 25 g total fat, 12 g saturated fat, 2 g fiber, 22 mg sodium

NOTE: If you prefer not to use alcohol, replace the orange liqueur with the same amount of fresh orange juice and ½ teaspoon almond extract instead of the amaretto.

ESPRESSO GRANITA WITH WHIPPED CREAM

Think of a granita as a slushie or Italian ice—except if you add alcohol to the recipe, it will be for adults only! You can easily multiply this recipe; just use a 9" x 13" baking dish for up to 6 cups of coffee. To lighten up the whipped cream, we've added a bit of reduced-fat sour cream. Its tartness balances out the bitter espresso—and saves 28 calories, 3 grams of total fat, and 2.5 grams of saturated fat.

PREP TIME: 10 MINUTES / TOTAL TIME: 3 HOURS 10 MINUTES / SERVES 8

- 2 cups hot espresso or very strong coffee
- ⅓ cup plus 1 tablespoon sugar
- 1½ teaspoons vanilla extract, divided
- ½ cup heavy whipping cream
- ½ cup reduced-fat sour cream
- 1 ounce bittersweet chocolate, shaved (optional)

1. In an 8" x 8" or 9" x 9" baking dish or nonreactive pan, gently stir together the espresso or coffee, ⅓ cup of the sugar, and 1 teaspoon of the vanilla until the sugar dissolves. Refrigerate until cool, about 30 minutes.

2. Freeze for 1 hour. Stir with a fork, scraping around the edges of the dish or pan. Freeze for an additional 2 to 2½ hours, scraping the granita and stirring the crystals into the center every 30 minutes to form icy flakes. The final mixture should not be slushy.

3. Before serving, in a small bowl using a whisk or an electric mixer, whip the heavy cream to stiff peaks. Add the sour cream, the remaining 1 tablespoon sugar, and the remaining ½ teaspoon vanilla. Continue to whip until creamy, 1 minute.

4. To serve, scoop ½ cup of granita into a bowl and dollop with 2 tablespoons cream. Shave chocolate on top, if using.

Per serving: 122 calories, 1 g protein, 13 g carbohydrates, 11 g sugars, 8 g total fat, 4.5 g saturated fat, 0 g fiber, 23 mg sodium

269

NOTE: Feel free to add a small splash of your favorite liqueur to the hot espresso or the whipped cream (or both!): Frangelico, Irish cream, Kahlúa, orange liqueur, even ouzo would complement the coffee flavor.

MERINGUES FOUR WAYS

These fluffy, chewy cookies can be infused with any flavor you like—but almond, cocoa, hazelnuts, and rosewater are especially mouthwatering. Bringing the egg whites to room temperature before beating them helps the stiff peaks form faster.

PREP TIME: 10 MINUTES / TOTAL TIME: 2 HOURS / SERVES 24 (3 PER SERVING)

MERINGUE BASE

3   egg whites, at room temperature
1   teaspoon vanilla extract
¼   teaspoon cream of tartar
    Pinch of kosher salt
⅔   cup sugar

ADDITIONS (CHOOSE ONE)

½   cup almonds, chopped
¼   cup cocoa
½   cup hazelnuts, chopped
1   teaspoon rosewater

1. Place the racks in the upper and lower third of the oven. Preheat the oven to 250°F. Line 2 baking sheets with parchment paper or silicone baking mats.

2. With an electric mixer on medium speed, beat the egg whites, vanilla, cream of tartar, and salt until foamy. Gradually add the sugar, mixing well between each addition to dissolve the sugar. Continue mixing until glossy stiff peaks form, about 5 minutes. Gently fold in your chosen addition.

3. Dollop spoonfuls of the batter onto the baking sheets, spacing them about 2" apart. Alter-natively, use a pastry bag or resealable plastic bag with the tip cut off to pipe the batter onto the sheets.

4. Bake until dry and firm to the touch, 40 to 45 minutes. Turn off the oven (do not open the oven door) and leave the meringues in the oven for 1 hour or up to overnight. Cool completely before storing in an airtight container at room temperature. The meringues are best if eaten within 5 days.

Per serving (base recipe): 24 calories, 1 g protein, 6 g carbohydrates, 6 g sugars, 0 g total fat, 0 g saturated fat, 0 g fiber, 13 mg sodium

Per serving (with ½ cup almonds): 35 calories, 1 g protein, 6 g carbohydrates, 6 g sugars, 1 g total fat, 0 g saturated fat, 0 g fiber, 13 mg sodium

Per serving (with ¼ cup cocoa): 26 calories, 1 g protein, 6 g carbohydrates, 6 g sugars, 0 g total fat, 0 g saturated fat, 0 g fiber, 13 mg sodium

Per serving (with ½ cup hazelnuts): 39 calories, 1 g protein, 6 g carbohydrates, 6 g sugars, 1 g total fat, 0 g saturated fat, 0 g fiber, 13 mg sodium

Per serving (with 1 teaspoon rosewater): 25 calories, 0 g protein, 6 g carbohydrates, 6 g sugars, 0 g total fat, 0 g saturated fat, 0 g fiber, 13 mg sodium

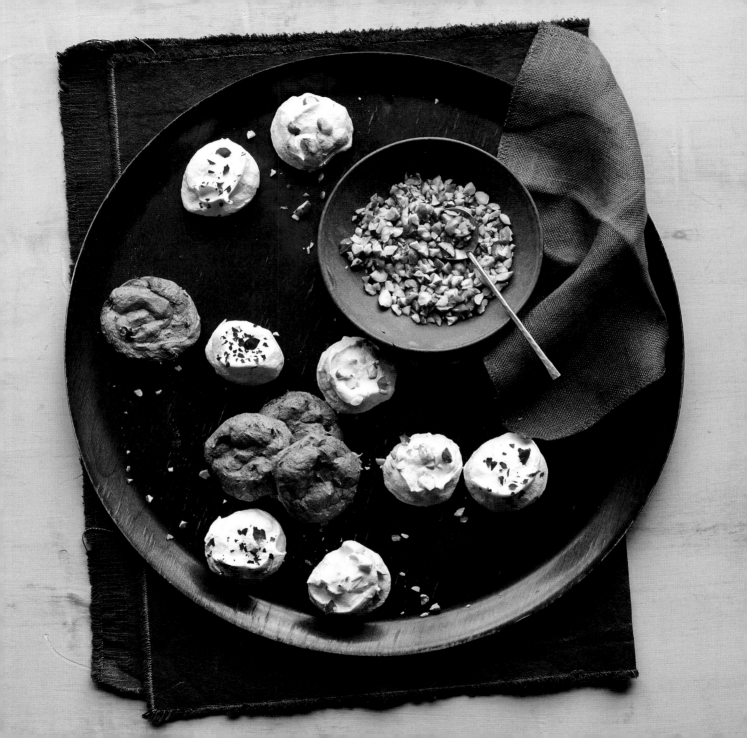

VEGAN MERINGUES FOUR WAYS

These vegan meringues are made with aquafaba—the liquid left over from canned beans. (Aqua is Latin for "water" and faba is Latin for "bean.") Aquafaba whips up just like egg whites—and believe it or not, makes for delicious vegan meringues. Give them a try!

PREP TIME: 5 MINUTES / TOTAL TIME: 3 HOURS / SERVES 24 (3 PER SERVING)

MERINGUE BASE

- 1 can (15 ounces) chickpeas
- 1 teaspoon vanilla extract
- ¼ teaspoon cream of tartar
- ¾ cup sugar

ADDITIONS (CHOOSE ONE)

- ½ cup almonds, chopped
- ¼ cup unsweetened cocoa
- ½ cup hazelnuts, chopped
- 1 teaspoon rosewater

1. Place the racks in the upper and lower third of the oven. Preheat the oven to 250°F. Line 2 baking sheets with parchment paper or silicone baking mats.

2. Drain the beans, reserving the liquid from the can. Reserve the beans themselves for another use.

3. In an electric stand mixer fitted with the whisk attachment, mix ½ cup of the aquafaba, the vanilla, and cream of tartar. Start on low, whip until frothy, and then increase to high. Mix until the mixture holds firm peaks, about 8 minutes.

4. With the mixer on high, gradually add the sugar, 1 tablespoon at a time. Scrape down the sides of the bowl once or twice. Keep whipping until smooth, firm peaks form, 8 to 10 minutes. Gently fold in your chosen additions.

5. Dollop spoonfuls of the batter onto the baking sheets, spacing them about 2" apart.

AQUAFABA

Aqua-huh? You may not be familiar with the name, but chances are you've dealt with this ingredient plenty of times. Aquafaba is the liquid left over from canned beans that most of us toss straight down the drain. But the thick, viscous texture and neutral flavor make it an ideal vegan substitute for eggs in meringues and other baked goods, dairy-free ice cream, and homemade mayonnaise and aioli. It might not be a traditional part of Mediterranean cooking, but if you're going to use canned chickpeas anyway, why let this versatile ingredient go to waste?

Alternatively, use a pastry bag or resealable plastic bag with the tip cut off to pipe the batter onto the sheets.

6. Bake until dry and firm to the touch, 1½ to 2 hours. Turn off the oven (do not open the oven door) and leave the meringues in the oven for 1 hour or up to overnight. Cool completely before storing in an airtight container at room temperature. The meringues are best if eaten within 3 days. They will begin to take on moisture as they sit and will become chewier and almost marshmallow-like.

Per serving (base recipe): 26 calories, 0 g protein, 6 g carbohydrates, 6 g sugars, 0 g total fat, 0 g saturated fat, 0 g fiber, 0 mg sodium

Per serving (with ½ cup almonds): 37 calories, 0 g protein, 7 g carbohydrates, 6 g sugars, 1 g total fat, 0 g saturated fat, 0 g fiber, 0 mg sodium

Per serving (with ¼ cup cocoa): 28 calories, 0 g protein, 7 g carbohydrates, 6 g sugars, 0 g total fat, 0 g saturated fat, 0 g fiber, 0 mg sodium

Per serving (with ½ cup hazelnuts): 41 calories, 0 g protein, 7 g carbohydrates, 6 g sugars, 1 g total fat, 0 g saturated fat, 0 g fiber, 0 mg sodium

Per serving (with 1 teaspoon rosewater): 27 calories, 0 g protein, 6 g carbohydrates, 6 g sugars, 0 g total fat, 0 g saturated fat, 0 g fiber, 0 mg sodium

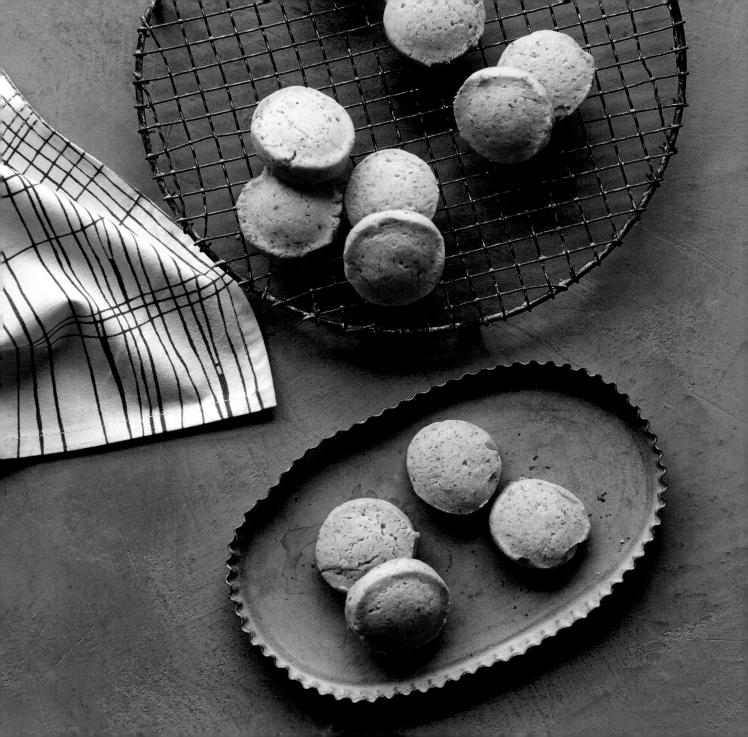

ORANGE-HAZELNUT OLIVE OIL COOKIES

These sweet, fragrant cookies get their rich, buttery texture from hazelnut and olive oil. They're a perfect treat for serving alongside coffee or tea.

PREP TIME: 10 MINUTES / TOTAL TIME: 2 HOURS 10 MINUTES / SERVES 24 (2 PER SERVING)

2 cups hazelnut flour (see note)
2¼ cups all-purpose flour
1 teaspoon baking powder
¼ teaspoon table salt
¾ cup sugar
½ cup extra-virgin olive oil
2 eggs
  Grated peel of 2 oranges
1 teaspoon vanilla extract

1. In a medium bowl, whisk together the flours, baking powder, and salt.

2. With an electric stand mixer on medium, combine the sugar, oil, eggs, orange peel, and vanilla. Increase the speed to medium high and mix until well combined, about 30 seconds. With the mixer on low speed, gradually add the dry ingredients and mix until the dough has just pulled together, 30 to 60 seconds.

3. Divide the dough in half. Pile one half of the dough onto a piece of parchment and form it into a log 11" long and 1½" in diameter. Wrap the parchment around the log and twist the ends to secure. Repeat with the remaining dough. Chill in the freezer until firm, about 1 hour.

4. Preheat the oven to 350°F. Line a baking sheet, or two depending on the size, with parchment paper or a silicone baking mat.

5. Unwrap one log of dough and cut into ½" slices. Place them on the baking sheets about 1" apart. Bake until golden on the bottoms and around the edges, about 15 minutes. Let cool completely on racks. Repeat with the remaining dough. The cookies will keep in an airtight container at room temperature for up to 1 week.

Per serving: 162 calories, 3 g protein, 14 g carbohydrates, 7 g sugars, 11 g total fat, 1.5 g saturated fat, 1 g fiber, 51 mg sodium

NOTE: If you can't get hazelnut flour, make your own from 2 cups toasted, skinned hazelnuts. Pulse them in a food processor until fine crumbs form. Do not overprocess, or you will end up with nut butter!

VANILLA-SAFFRON SEMIFREDDO

This creamy Italian dessert is like a frozen mousse. Its name means "half cold," which is appropriate since it never fully freezes. It's surprisingly airy, given its base of cream, sugar, and eggs. We've lightened it up a smidge and simplified it by removing the egg-white meringue that's frequently folded in.

PREP TIME: 5 MINUTES / TOTAL TIME: 30 MINUTES + FREEZING TIME / SERVES 12

Generous pinch of saffron (about 20 threads)
⅓ cup sugar
3 egg yolks, room temperature
½ teaspoon vanilla bean paste or the seeds of ½ vanilla bean
1½ cups cold heavy cream
1 pint fresh raspberries, for serving

1. Line the 12 cups of a muffin pan individually with plastic wrap. Prepare an ice bath by filling a large bowl with ice water.

2. Set a medium glass bowl over a pot of simmering water (the bottom of the bowl should not touch the water). Add the saffron and cook, stirring constantly to break up the threads, until fragrant, 2 to 3 minutes.

3. Add the sugar, egg yolks, and vanilla, whisking to combine. Whisk constantly, or beat with a hand mixer, until the yolks are pale yellow and tripled in volume, about 5 minutes.

4. Transfer the bowl to the ice bath and chill, whisking occasionally, until cool, about 3 minutes.

5. Meanwhile, in a large bowl with a hand mixer or an electric stand mixer on medium, whip the cream until stiff peaks form, 2 to 3 minutes.

6. Gently whisk ⅓ of the whipped cream into the cooled egg mixture until smooth. Fold in the remaining cream with a spatula until just incorporated.

7. Pour ¼ cup of the mixture into each muffin cup and smooth over the tops with an offset spatula. Do not tap the muffin tin on the counter to help spread out the mixture, as that will deflate it. Lay a sheet of plastic wrap over the tops of all the cups and freeze overnight.

8. To serve, use the plastic wrap to remove 1 cup from the muffin tin. Invert onto a small plate or into a bowl and peel off the wrap from the bottom. Scatter the raspberries around the semifrozen cup.

Per serving: 150 calories, 2 g protein, 9 g carbohydrates, 7 g sugars, 12 g total fat, 7.5 g saturated fat, 1 g fiber, 14 mg sodium

NOTE: Warm a spatula under hot tap water, wipe it off, and run it over the tops of the semifreddo cups once they're unmolded to smooth them. The crinkles from the plastic wrap will disappear.

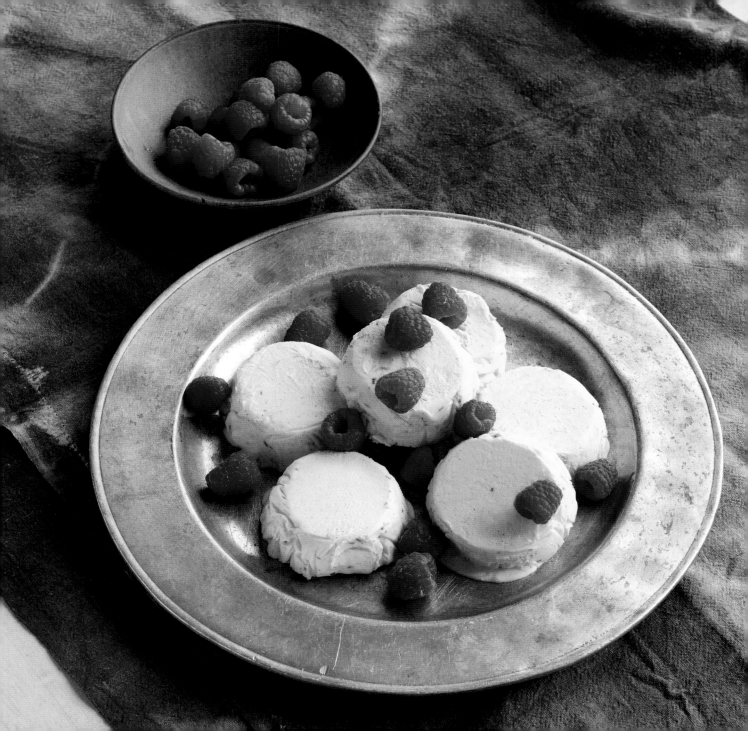

SAMPLE MENUS

WEEKEND BRUNCH
Italian Vegetable Frittata (page 70)
Blueberry-Lemon Tea Cakes (page 77)
Homemade Ricotta Cheese and Breakfast Bowl
   (page 74)
Fresh seasonal fruit

PICNIC LUNCH
Mediterranean Niçoise Salad (page 108)
Fried Baby Artichokes with Lemon-Garlic Aioli
   (page 160), served at room temperature
Hummus (page 149) with Whole Wheat Pitas
   (page 164)
Quince Paste (page 261), served with
   Manchego cheese

SIMPLE WEEKDAY LUNCHES
Arugula Salad with Grapes, Goat Cheese,
   and Za'atar Croutons (page 107)
Baba Ghanoush (page 154) with Whole Wheat
   Pitas (page 164)
Cranberry Bean Minestrone (page 93)

Crusty whole grain bread
Fresh seasonal fruit
Kidney Bean Peasant Salad (page 131)
Cheese-Stuffed Dates (page 167)

SIMPLE WEEKDAY DINNERS
Grilled Rosemary-Lemon Turkey Cutlets (page 231)
Wild Greens Salad with Fresh Herbs (page 111)
Crusty whole grain bread
Strawberry Mascarpone Parfaits (page 268)
Orecchiette with Broccoli Rabe and Anchovies
   (page 215)
Greek Salad with Lemon-Oregano Vinaigrette
   (page 105)
Baked Red Snapper with Potatoes and Tomatoes
   (page 243)
Pear-Fennel Salad with Pomegranate (page 125)
Meringues (page 270) made with almonds

278

SUNDAY DINNER

Roast Pork Loin with Juniper Berries and Honey
(page 244)

Spinach Salad with Pomegranate, Lentils, and
Pistachios (page 112)

Saffron Couscous with Almonds, Currants, and
Scallions (page 180)

Vanilla Saffron Semifreddo (page 276)

MEZE MEAL

Halloumi, Watermelon, Tomato Kebabs with Basil
Oil Drizzle (page 171)

Arnabit (*Roasted Cauliflower*) with Spicy Tahini
Sauce (page 177)

Crispy Spiced Chickpeas (page 152)

Mixed-Olive Tapenade (page 163) with whole
grain toasts

Vegetarian Dolmades (*Stuffed Grape Leaves*),
(page 147)

VEGETARIAN FEAST

Kushari (*Egyptian Rice, Lentils, and Ditalini*),
(page 217)

Turkish Red Lentil Bride Soup (page 102)

Roasted Cauliflower "Steak" Salad (page 116)

Tahini Baklava Cups (page 257)

SOUP NIGHT

Harira (*Moroccan Chickpea and Lentil Soup*),
(page 98)

Red Pepper, Pomegranate, and Walnut Salad
(page 115)

Pear and Cardamom Sorbet (page 265)

BACKYARD BARBECUE BASH

Turkey Burgers with Feta and Dill (page 140)

Grilled Halloumi with Mixed Grilled Vegetables
(page 127)

Bravas-Style Potatoes (page 155)

Turkish Shepherd's Salad (page 133)

Almond-Peach Ice Pops (page 267)

279

ENDNOTES

INTRODUCTION

1   Renna M et al., "The Mediterranean diet between traditional foods and human health: The culinary example of Puglia (Southern Italy)," *International Journal of Gastronomy and Food Science* 2 (2015): 63–71.

CHAPTER I

1   Estruch R et al., "Primary prevention of cardiovascular disease with a Mediterranean Diet," *New England Journal of Medicine* 368 (2013): 1279–90.

2   "Mediterranean diet: A heart-healthy eating plan," Mayo Clinic, accessed March 24, 2017, mayoclinic.org/healthy -lifestyle/nutrition-and-healthy-eating/in-depth /mediterranean-diet/art-20047801?pg=1.

3   Bonaccio M et al., "Mediterranean diet and low-grade subclinical inflammation: the Moli-sani study," *Endocrine, Metabolic & Immune Disorders—Drug Targets* 15, no. 1 (2015): 18–24.

4   Brill J, "The Mediterranean diet and your health," *American Journal of Lifestyle Medicine* 3, no. 1 (2009): 44–56.

5   "Mediterranean diet pyramid," Oldways, accessed March 1, 2017, oldwayspt.org/traditional-diets/mediterranean-diet.

6   Katz D et al., "Can we say what diet is best for health?," *Annual Review of Public Health* 35 (2014): 83–103.

7   McLaren DS, "The kingdom of the Keyses," *Nutrition* 13 (1993): 249–53.

8   Tong T et al., "Prospective association of the Mediterranean diet with cardiovascular disease incidence and mortality and its population impact in a non-Mediterranean population: The EPIC-Norfolk study," *BMC Medicine* 14 (2016): 135.

9   Stewart R et al., "Dietary patterns and the risk of major adverse cardiovascular events in a global study of high-risk patients with stable coronary heart disease," *European Heart Journal* 37, no. 25 (2016): 1993–2001.

10 Estruch R et al., "Primary prevention of cardiovascular disease with a Mediterranean diet," *New England Journal of Medicine* 368 (2013): 1279–90.

11 Yusuf S et al., "Blood-pressure and cholesterol lowering in persons without cardiovascular disease," *New England Journal of Medicine* 374 (2016): 2032–43.

12 Babio N et al., "Mediterranean diets and metabolic syndrome status in the PREDIMED randomized trial," *Canadian Medical Association Journal* 186, no. 17 (2014): E649–57.

13 Mancini J et al., "Systematic review of the Mediterranean diet for long-term weight loss," *American Journal of Medicine* 129 (2016): 407–15.

14 Mancini J et al., "Systematic review of the Mediterranean diet for long term weight loss," *American Journal of Medicine* 129 (2016): 407–15.

15 "Children consuming a Mediterranean Diet are 15% less likely to be overweight," Sahlgrenska Academy, University of Gothenburg, June, 10, 2014, accessed February 10, 2017, sahlgrenska.gu.se/english/research/news-events/news-article//children-consuming-a-mediterranean-diet-are-15--less-likely-to-be-overweight-.cid1222759.

16 Estruch R et al., "Effect of a high-fat Mediterranean diet on bodyweight and waist circumference: A prespecified secondary outcomes analysis of the PREDIMED randomised control trial," *Lancet Diabetes & Endocrinology* 4, no. 8 (2016): 666–76.

17 Koloverou E et al., "The effect of Mediterranean diet on the development of type 2 diabetes mellitus: A meta-analysis of 10 prospective studies and 136,846 participants," *Metabolism* 63, no. 7 (2014): 903–11.

18 Schwingshackl L et al., "Does a Mediterranean-type diet reduce cancer risk?," *Current Nutrition Reports* 5 (2016): 9–17.

19 Biasini C et al., "Mediterranean diet influences breast cancer relapse: Preliminary results of the SETA PROJECT," *Journal of Clinical Oncology* 34 (2016): e13039.

20 Luciano M et al., "Mediterranean-type diet and brain structural change from 73 to 76 years in a Scottish cohort," *Neurology* 88, no. 5 (2017): 449–55.

21 Clare M et al., "MIND diet associated with reduced incidence of Alzheimer's disease," *Alzheimer's & Dementia* 11, no. 9 (2015): 1007–14.

22 Hardman J et al., "Adherence to a Mediterranean-style diet and effects on cognition in adults: A qualitative evaluation and systematic review of longitudinal and prospective trials," *Frontiers in Nutrition* 3, no. 22 (2016): 1–13.

23 Trichopoulou A et al., "Anatomy of health effects of Mediterranean diet: Greek EPIC prospective cohort study," *British Medical Journal* 338 (2009): b2337.

24 Crous-Bou M et al., "Mediterranean diet and telomere length in Nurses' Health Study: Population based cohort study," *British Medical Journal* 349 (2014): g6674.

25 Jacka F et al., "Association of western and traditional diets with depression and anxiety in women," *American Journal of Psychiatry* 167 (2010): 1–7.

26 Jacka F et al., "A randomised controlled trial of dietary improvement for adults with major depression (the 'SMILES' trial)," *BMC Medicine* 15 (2017): 23.

27 Woolley K et al., "A recipe for friendship: Similar food consumption promotes trust and cooperation," *Journal of Consumer Psychology* 27, no. 1 (2017): 1–10.

281

28 Kawachi I et al., "Social ties and mental health," *Journal of Urban Health* 78, no. 3 (2001): 458–67.

29 "The biology of emotion—and what it may teach us about helping people live longer," Harvard T.H. Chan School of Public Health, Harvard University, accessed February 10, 2017, hsph.harvard.edu/news/magazine/happiness-stress -heart-disease.

30 Katz D et al., "Can we say what diet is best for health?," *Annual Review of Public Health* 35 (2014): 83–103.

31 Higgins J et al., "Resistant starch consumption promotes lipid oxidation," *Nutrition & Metabolism* 1 (2004): 8.

32 Bodinham C et al., "Acute ingestion of resistant starch reduces food intake in healthy adults," *British Journal of Nutrition* 103 (2010): 917–22.

33 De Filippis F et al., "High level adherence to a Mediterranean diet beneficially impacts the gut microbiota and associated metabolome," *Gut* 65, no. 11 (2015): 1812–21.

34 Carlsen MH et al., "The total antioxidant content of more than 3,100 foods, beverages, spices, herbs, and supplements used worldwide," *Nutrition Journal* 9 (2010): 3.

35 Ibid.

36 Li D et al., "Health benefits of anthocyanins and molecular mechanisms: Update from recent decade," *Critical Reviews in Food Science and Nutrition* 57, no. 8 (2017): 1729–41.

37 "Vitamin C," Linus Pauling Institute, Oregon State University, accessed March 27, 2017, lpi.oregonstate.edu /mic/vitamins/vitamin-C.

38 "Lutein & Zeaxanthin," American Optometric Association, accessed March 27, 2017, aoa.org/patients-and-public /caring-for-your-vision/diet-and-nutrition/lutein?sso=y.

39 "Beta-carotene," University of Maryland Medical Center, accessed March 24, 2017, umm.edu/health/medical /altmed/supplement/betacarotene.

40 "Quercetin," University of Maryland Medical Center, accessed March 24, 2017, umm.edu/health/medical/altmed /supplement/quercetin.

41 Vinson J et al., "Nuts, especially walnuts, have both antioxidant quantity and efficacy and exhibit significant potential health benefits," *Food & Function* 3 (2012): 134–40.

42 Renna M et al., "The Mediterranean diet between traditional foods and human health: The culinary example of Puglia (Southern Italy)," *International Journal of Gastronomy and Food Science* 2 (2015): 63–71.

43 Alexander D et al., "A meta-analysis of randomized controlled trials and prospective cohort studies of eicosapentaenoic and docosahexaenoic long-chain omega-3 fatty acids and coronary heart disease risk," *Mayo Clinic Proceedings* 92, no. 1 (2017): 15–29.

44 Chen M et al., "Dairy fat and risk of cardiovascular disease in 3 cohorts of US adults," *American Journal of Clinical Nutrition.* 14, no. 5 (2016): 1209–17.

45 Kratz M et al., "The relationship between high-fat dairy consumption and obesity, cardiovascular, and metabolic disease," *European Journal of Nutrition* 52, no. 1 (2013): 1–24.

46 Zheng H et al., "Metabolomics investigation to shed light on cheese as a possible piece in the French paradox puzzle," *Journal of Agricultural and Food Chemistry* 63:10 (2015): 2830–39.

47 "Common questions about contaminants in seafood," Environmental Defense Fund Seafood Selector, accessed March 24, 2017, seafood.edf.org/common-questions-about -contaminants-seafood.

48 "PCBs in fish and shellfish," Environmental Defense Fund Seafood Selector, accessed February 10, 2017, seafood.edf .org/pcbs-fish-and-shellfish.

49 Zong G et al., "Intake of individual saturated fatty acids and risk of coronary heart disease in US men and women: Two prospective longitudinal cohort studies," *British Medical Journal* 355 (2016): i5796.

50 "Processed foods: what's okay and what to avoid," Academy of Nutrition and Dietetics, accessed March 25, 2017, eatright.org/resource/food/nutrition/nutrition-facts-and -food-labels/avoiding-processed-foods.

51 Mozaffarian D et al., "Changes in diet and lifestyle and long-term weight gain in women and men," *New England Journal of Medicine* 364 (2011): 2392–404.

52 Cornill Y et al., "Pleasure as an ally of healthy eating? Contrasting visceral and Epicurean eating pleasure and their association with portion size preferences and wellbeing," *Appetite* 104 (2016): 52–59.

CHAPTER 2

1 Moore L et al., "Adults meeting fruit and vegetable intake recommendations—United States, 2013," *Morbidity and Mortality Weekly Report* 64, no. 26 (2015): 709–28.

2 "Why should I limit sodium?" American Heart Association, accessed March 24, 2017, heart.org/idc/groups/heart-public/@wcm/@hcm/documents/downloadable/ucm_300625.pdf.

3 "Added sugars," American Heart Association, accessed March 24, 2017, heart.org/HEARTORG/HealthyLiving/HealthyEating/Nutrition/Added-Sugars_UCM_305858_Article.jsp#.WNV2JRiZNAY.

4 Swithers S, "Artificial sweeteners produce the counterintuitive effect of inducing metabolic derangements," *Trends in Endocrinology and Metabolism* 24, no. 9 (2013): 431–41.

5 "Red wine and resveratrol: good for your heart?," Mayo Clinic, accessed February 17, 2017, mayoclinic.org/diseases-conditions/heart-disease/in-depth/red-wine/art-20048281.

6 Toledo E et al., "Mediterranean diet and invasive breast cancer risk among women at high cardiovascular risk in the PREDIMED trial: A randomized clinical trial," *JAMA Internal Medicine* 175, no. 11 (2015): 1752–60.

7 Zhang SM et al., "Plasma folate, vitamin B6, vitamin B12, homocysteine, and risk of breast cancer," *Journal of the National Cancer Institute* 5, no. 95 (2003): 373–80.

8 Baranski M et al., "Higher antioxidant and lower cadmium concentrations and lower incidence of pesticide residues in organically grown crops: A systematic literature review and meta-analyses," *British Journal of Nutrition* 112, no. 5 (2014): 794–811.

9 Reganold J et al., "Fruit and soil quality of organic and conventional strawberry agroecosystems," *PLOS ONE* 5, no. 9 (2010): e12346.

10 "Organic foods: What you need to know about eating organic," Helpguide.org, accessed March 27, 2017, helpguide.org/articles/healthy-eating/organic-foods.htm.

11 Flynn M et al., "Economical healthy diets (2012): Including lean animal protein costs more than using extra virgin olive oil," *Journal of Hunger & Environmental Nutrition* 10, no. 4 (2015): 1–16.

CHAPTER 3

1 Suez J et al., "Artificial sweeteners induce glucose intolerance by altering the gut microbiota," *Nature* 514, no. 7521 (2014): 181–86.

2 "Trans fats," American Heart Association, accessed March 25, 2017, heart.org/HEARTORG/HealthyLiving/HealthyEating/Nutrition/Trans-Fats_UCM_301120_Article.jsp#.WNZxXRiZNAY.

3 "Final determination regarding partially hydrogenated oils (removing trans fat)," US Food & Drug Administration, accessed March 25, 2017, fda.gov/Food/IngredientsPackagingLabeling/FoodAdditivesIngredients/ucm449162.htm.

4 "WHO report says eating processed meat is carcinogenic: Understanding the findings," Harvard T.H. Chan School of Public Health, accessed March 25, 2017, hsph.harvard.edu/nutritionsource/2015/11/03/report-says-eating-processed-meat-is-carcinogenic-understanding-the-findings.

5 "EWG's Dirty Dozen Guide to Food Additives: Generally recognized as safe—but is it?," Environmental Working Group, accessed March 25, 2017, ewg.org/research/ewg-s-dirty-dozen-guide-food-additives/generally-recognized-as-safe-but-is-it.

6 "Potassium bromate," National Institute for Occupational Safety and Health, Centers for Disease Control and Prevention, accessed March 25, 2017, cdc.gov/niosh/ipcsneng/neng1115.html.

7 "Food dyes: A rainbow of risks," Center for Science in the Public Interest, accessed March 25, 2017, cspinet.org/resource/food-dyes-rainbow-risks.

8 Smith T et al., "Caramel color in soft drinks and exposure to 4-methylimidazole: A quantitative risk assessment," *PLOS ONE* 10, no. 2 (2015): e0118138.

9 Baad-Hansen L et al., "Effect of systemic monosodium glutamate (MSG) on headache and pericranial muscle sensitivity," *Cephalalgia* 30, no. 1 (2010): 68–76.

10 Piqueras-Fiszman B et al., "The weight of the container influences expected satiety, perceived density, and subsequent expected fullness," *Appetite* 58, no. 2 (2012): 559–62.

11 Martin-Biggers J et al., "Come and get it! A discussion of family mealtime literature and factors affecting obesity risk," *Advances in Nutrition* 5 (2014): 235–47.

12 Cook E et al., "Do family meals really make a difference?," College of Human Ecology, Department of Policy Analysis and Management, Cornell University, accessed February 2, 2017, human.cornell.edu/pam/outreach/upload/Family-Mealtimes-2.pdf.

13 Wansink B et al., "The clean plate club: About 92% of self-served food is eaten," *International Journal of Obesity* 39 (2015): 371–74.

14 Loucks E et al., "Associations of dispositional mindfulness with obesity and central adiposity: The New England Family Study," *International Journal of Behavioral Medicine* 23, no. 2 (2016): 224–33.

15 Loucks E et al., "Positive associations of dispositional mindfulness with cardiovascular health: The New England Family Study," *International Journal of Behavioral Medicine* 22, no. 4 (2015): 540–50.

16 Loucks E et al., "Associations of mindfulness with glucose regulation and diabetes," *American Journal of Health Behavior* 40, no. 2 (2016): 258–67.

17 van der Wal R et al., "Leaving a flat taste in your mouth: Task load reduces taste perception," *Psychological Science* 24, no. 7 (2013): 1277–84.

18 Vohs K et al., "Rituals enhance consumption," *Psychological Science* 24, no. 9 (2013): 1714–21.

19 Richardson C et al., "A meta-analysis of pedometer-based walking interventions and weight loss," *Annals of Family Medicine* 6, no. 1 (2008): 69–77.

CHAPTER 4

1 Ogden J et al., "Distraction, restrained eating and disinhibition: An experimental study of food intake and the impact of 'eating on the go,'" *Journal of Health Psychology* 22, no. 1 (2017): 39–50.

2 Clodoveo M et al., "In the ancient world, virgin olive oil was called 'liquid gold' by Homer and 'the great healer' by Hippocrates. Why has this mythic image been forgotten?," *Food Research International* 62 (2014): 1062–68.

3 Estruch R et al., "Primary prevention of cardiovascular disease with a Mediterranean diet," *New England Journal of Medicine* 368, no. 14 (2013): 1279–90.

4 Charles R et al., "Protection from hypertension in mice by the Mediterranean diet is mediated by nitro fatty acid inhibition of soluble epoxide hydrolase," *Proceedings of the National Academy of Sciences of the United States of America* 111, no. 22 (2014): 8167–72.

5 Abuznait A et al., "Olive-oil-derived oleocanthal enhances ß-amyloid clearance as a potential neuroprotective mechanism," *ACS Chemical Neuroscience* 4, no. 6 (2013): 973–82.

6 "Olive oil makes you feel full," Technical University of Munich, accessed February 27, 2017, tum.de/en/about-tum/news/press-releases/detail/article/30517.

7 Zamroziewicz M et al. "Parahippocampal cortex mediates the relationship between lutein and crystallized intelligence in healthy, older adults." *Frontiers in Aging Neuroscience* 8:297 (2016).

8 "Eating green leafy vegetables keeps mental abilities sharp." Federation of American Societies for Experimental Biology (FASEB), accessed February 28, 2017, http://www.newswise.com/articles/eating-green-leafy-vegetables-keeps-mental-abilities-sharp.

CHAPTER 5

1 "Foods that fight cancer: Grapes and grape juice," American Institute for Cancer Research, accessed February 27, 2017, aicr.org/foods-that-fight-cancer/foodsthatfightcancer_grapes_and_grape_juice.html.

2 Chen GC et al., "Cheese consumption and risk of cardiovascular disease: A meta-analysis of prospective studies," *European Journal of Nutrition* (August 2016): doi:10.1007/s00394-016-1292-z.

3 de Goede J et al., "Dairy consumption and risk of stroke: A systematic review and updated dose-response meta-analysis of prospective cohort studies," *Journal of the American Heart Association* 5, no. 5 (2016): e002787.

4 Gazan R et al., "Dietary patterns in the French adult population: A study from the second French national cross-sectional dietary survey (INCA2) (2006–2007)," *British*

Journal of Nutrition 116 (2016): 300–315.

5   Mozaffarian D et al., "Trans-palmitoleic acid, metabolic risk factors, and new-onset diabetes in U.S. adults: A cohort study," *Annals of Internal Medicine* 153, no. 12 (2010): 790–99.

6   Reid K et al., "Effect of garlic on serum lipids: An updated meta-analysis," *Nutrition Reviews* 71, no. 5 (2013): 282–99.

CHAPTER 6

1   Kristensen M et al., "Meals based on vegetable protein sources (beans and peas) are more satiating than meals based on animal protein sources (veal and pork)—A randomized cross-over meal test study," *Food & Nutrition Research* 60, no. 1 (2017): 1654–61.

2   Kim S et al., "Effects of dietary pulse consumption on body weight: A systematic review and meta-analysis of randomized controlled trials," *American Journal of Clinical Nutrition* 103 (2016): 1213–23.

3   Song M et al., "Association of animal and plant protein intake with all-cause and cause-specific mortality," *JAMA Internal Medicine* 176, no. 10 (2016): 1453–63.

4   "Does grape juice offer the same heart benefits as red wine?," Mayo Clinic, accessed March 25, 2017, mayoclinic.org/healthy-lifestyle/nutrition-and-healthy-eating/expert-answers/food-and-nutrition/faq-20058529.

5   Cassidy A et al., "High anthocyanin intake is associated with a reduced risk of myocardial infarction in young and middle-aged women," *Circulation* 127 (2013): 188–96.

6   Karl JP et al., "Substituting whole grains for refined grains in a 6-wk randomized trial favorably affects energy-balance metrics in healthy men and postmenopausal women," *American Journal of Clinical Nutrition* 105, no. 3 (2017): 589–99.

7   Chen M et al., "Dairy consumption and risk of type 2 diabetes: 3 cohorts of US adults and an updated meta-analysis," *BMC Medicine* 12 (2014): 215.

CHAPTER 7

1   Roe L et al., "Salad and satiety: The effect of timing of salad consumption on meal energy intake," *Appetite* 58, no. 1 (2012): 242–48.

2   Flood JE et al., "Soup preloads in a variety of forms reduce meal energy intake," *Appetite* 49, no. 3 (2007): 626–34.

3   Zu K et al., "Dietary lycopene, angiogenesis, and prostate cancer: A prospective study in the prostate-specific antigen era," *Journal of the National Cancer Institute* 106, no. 2 (2014): djt430.

4   Li X et al., "Dietary and circulating lycopene and stroke risk: A meta-analysis of prospective studies," *Scientific Reports* 4 (2014): 5031.

5   Mozaffarian D et al., "Fish intake, contaminants, and human health: Evaluating the risks and benefits," *JAMA* 296, no. 15 (2006): 1885–99.

6   "Is there any benefit to taking fish oil supplements for depression?," Mayo Clinic, accessed February 27, 2017, mayoclinic.org/diseases-conditions/depression/expert-answers/fish-oil-supplements/faq-20058143.

7   Corder R et al., "Oenology: Red wine procyanidins and vascular health," *Nature* 444, no. 30 (2006): 566.

8   Gepner Y et al., "Two-year moderate alcohol intervention in adults with type 2 diabetes: A 2-year randomized, controlled trial," *Annals of Internal Medicine* 163, no. 8 (2015): 569–79.

9   di Giuseppe R et al., "Alcohol consumption and n-3 polyunsaturated fatty acids in healthy men and women from 3 European populations," *American Journal of Clinical Nutrition* 89 (2009): 354–62.

10 Smith JS et al., "Effect of marinades on the formation of heterocyclic amines in grilled beef steaks," *Journal of Food Science* 73, no. 6 (2008): 100–105.

11 "Beta-carotene," University of Maryland Medical Center, accessed March 24, 2017, umm.edu/health/medical/altmed/supplement/betacarotene.

CHAPTER 8

1   Khalil M et al., "The potential role of honey and its polyphenols in preventing heart diseases: A review," *African Journal of Traditional, Complementary, and Alternative Medicines* 7, no. 4 (2010): 315–21.

2   Asama T et al., "Lactobacillus kunkeei YB38 from honeybee products enhances IgA production in healthy adults," *Journal of Applied Microbiology* 119, no. 3 (2015): 818–26.

3   Schmidt K et al., "Prebiotic intake reduces the waking cortisol response and alters emotional bias in healthy volunteers," *Psychopharmacology* 232, no. 10 (2015): 1793–1801.

4   "Comparison of vitamin, mineral and antioxidant levels in raw and processed honey," Ropa Science Research, the National Honey Board, accessed January 27, 2017, honey.com/images/uploads/general/Nutritional_Analysis _Raw_vs_Processed_Honey-102912.pdf.

5   "Vitamin C and skin health," Linus Pauling Institute, Oregon State University, accessed March 25, 2017, lpi. oregonstate.edu/mic/health-disease/skin-health /vitamin-C.

6   Bao Y et al., "Association of nut consumption with total and cause-specific mortality," *New England Journal of Medicine* 369, no. 21 (2013): 2001–2011.

7   Ibid.

8   Tan S et al., "A review of the effects of nuts on appetite, food intake, metabolism, and body weight," *American Journal of Clinical Nutrition* 100 (2014): 412S–22S.

9   Kris-Etherton P, "Walnuts decrease risk of cardiovascular disease: A summary of efficacy and biologic mechanisms," *Journal of Nutrition* 144 (2014): 547S–54S.

10 Bertoia M et al., "Changes in intake of fruits and vegetables and weight change in United States men and women followed for up to 24 years: Analysis from three prospective cohort studies," *PLOS Medicine* 12, no. 9 (2015): e1001878.

ENDNOTES

INDEX

288

INDEX

290

291

292

293

294